Pain-Free
Massage Therapist

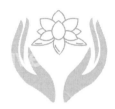

The common sense way to make you a
pain-free, durable, and productive
massage therapist.

Mark E. Liskey,
LMT, CNMT

Library of Congress Cataloging-In-Publication Data

Names: Liskey, Mark, author.

Title: The Pain-Free Massage Therapist: The Common Sense Way to Make You a Pain-Free, Durable and Productive Massage Therapist/ Mark Liskey

Description: 1st edition. | Phoenixville, PA: Mark Liskey, [2021] |

Includes bibliographical references.

ISBN 978-1-7375265-0-6

Dedication

To Lisa, my wife, editor, coach and advisor.
Your love, determination, and persistence has
made all the difference. Without you there
would be no book.

Table of Contents

Forward

Let's just say that I was not an early adopter of Mark's work. I'm a rule-following people-pleaser who didn't want to give up the thumb-killing moves that made my clients groan with pleasure. I didn't want anything to do with massage tools ("pokey sticks" as I called them), and I certainly didn't want to feel awkward doing any weird leaning stuff. Every piece of resistance Mark has ever encountered on this subject, he heard from me first. (I'm *that* wife.) Ultimately though, I couldn't argue with his results.

I saw him fifteen years ago when he was on the verge of ending his massage career due to pain. I see him now, almost 30 years into his career, still able to do up to 30 massages a week (many of them deep pressure massages) without pain. I watched the transformation unfold.

He was in pain. Now he isn't.

It was the principles and techniques in this book that were responsible for that change. It's that simple.

I'm a believer now, for sure. If pain is threatening the massage career you love, or if you're hoping to avoid ever being in that situation, I believe experimenting with and mastering some of the ideas in this book can help you too. Here's to being a pain-free massage therapist!

Lisa Westfall, LMT

Preface:
You Can Massage Pain-Free

The first conversation that I had with a massage therapist didn't go well. I was 20-something, working out like crazy, and was dinged up with some overuse injuries.

I really wanted to try massage, but massage in the 1980s wasn't main stream, and finding a legitimate massage person in the Philadelphia, PA suburbs required some work.

At the time I had a gardening business and a client recommended Brenda. I trusted the client. So, why not call?

When I did, let's just say it was an interesting conversation.

Brenda, speaking in a thick Slavic accent, was annoyed.

"Who is this?", she demanded.

Mark Liskey, I said.

"Who gave you my number?"

Juanita Simpson.

"What do you want?"

A massage.

"Ugh. I have seven massages tomorrow. Six on Saturday. My God! My hands! You have to have massage?"

I thiiink so…

There were sounds of Brenda looking through her schedule book, then she barked: "What's wrong with you?"

My knee is bothering me.

"What else?"

Well, my back hurts some.

"That's it?"

I guess.

"You can wait. Call back in two months."

Click.

No joke. Brenda chased me away.

It's not surprising that this conversation pops up in my mind whenever I experience pain from doing massage. Massage is physical work. If you do massage for any length of time, you *will* experience a Brenda moment. My Brenda moment was actually a Brenda year.

Time to Hang Up My Hands?

It was June of 2013, and I was sweating bullets. I had severe pain in my neck, shoulder and arm, and I got some seriously bad news at the orthopedist's office.

An old football injury, compounded by years of working out and lots of massage, left me with a banged up left shoulder joint, cervical radiculopathy and cubital tunnel syndrome.

"Find a new career," said Dr. That's-Easy-For-You-To-Say.

I was no stranger to being in pain from doing massage. Early on in my massage career, I was blowing out my thumbs because of all the detail work I was doing. Why all the detail work? I was certified in and practicing neuromuscular therapy (NMT).

One NMT concept is that you must work the origin, insertion and body of the muscle for the best release. As thorough a massage as this was for the client, it was equally thorough in beating up the MT's hands.

I guess I should have seen this coming. When I was going through the NMT program I would do exchanges with my friend Maggie, who was also going through the program with me. One day she walked in with all her distal finger joints taped. She looked like she could have been in the *Spirit of 76* Revolutionary War painting next to the fife player with the head-bandage.

I'm not knocking NMT. It was a comprehensive program that launched my massage career, but it was almost entirely client-centric, meaning it was focused on the client's well-being, with little attention given to the therapist's durability.

NMT was not alone in this category. Pfrimmer had a reputation of sending MTs into a very early retirement because the techniques severely stressed the practitioner's hands. And sacrificing your hands to get the job done didn't seem to be exclusively an American idea either.

Once an acupuncturist from China who I shared office space with told me that I should learn the Chinese massage he did because it was so much superior to the massage I did.

I said, "Okay, can you show me some techniques?"

No.

Initially, I was ticked because I thought he was withholding information that could help me be a better therapist. But as the conversation went on, he eventually confessed that the massage he did—that was so superior to my massage—hurt his hands way too much for him to show me.

Did you catch the operative word? "Did." As in, past tense. His superior techniques hurt him so much he could no longer do them.

The message to me continued to be that in order to be a rock-star MT, you needed to kill your hands.

When I look around at new MTs coming into the business today, I don't think the idea of sacrificing your body to do your job has gone away. It's an idea that when you look at it more closely, doesn't make a lot of sense.

Granted, you sometimes have to do things that make your body temporarily uncomfortable to get the job done. But if you're consistently and blindly throwing a body part into harm's way, you're not going to last. And you're going to start resenting your work and your clients.

I know this is a widespread problem in our industry. How do I know? Because you tell me. Every time I meet a new class of CE students, I hear their stories. Well, not at first. At first, everyone has their "Massage Therapist Super Hero" façade up. But as the class goes on, the façade starts to crumble, and the truth comes out that many of them work in pain.

The evidence is overwhelming when I think about my practice. I've accumulated a lot of MT clients who come see me for neck, shoulder, arm, hand and back pain issues. Why? Because massage hurts them. And on my blog site, MTs from around the world constantly email me asking for help. So I know.

But back when I was practicing NMT, I didn't know all that yet. I just knew that I hurt and something needed to change.

Fortunately for me, I had an entry point for experimenting with ways to massage in less pain. NMT was big on massage tools, like the T-bar.

The T-bar Paradox

The T-bar is a simple tool, shaped like a T with a plastic or rubber tip.

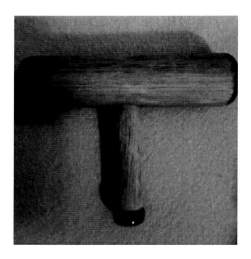

(P1)

The function of the T-bar in NMT is to help the MT reach and apply pressure to muscle attachments and hard to reach places. A byproduct of using a T-bar was that it could be a thumb replacement.

In other words, get the spot with the T-bar and if it helped your thumbs, great. If not, oh well.

Eventually, my "sacrificing your body to get the job done" mindset started to crack because the longer I did NMT and the more clients I saw, the more the T-bar hurt my fingers.

There's an easy explanation for why the T-bar hurt my fingers. In NMT we were taught to grip the tip of the T-bar to control it, sort of the way you hold a pen or pencil.

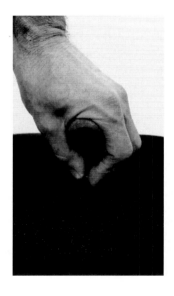

(P2)

That gripping put serious stress in the 1st, 2nd and 3rd distal finger joints. A little gripping—a light client-load for the day—was okay. But if I had a normal or heavy client-load for the day, my fingers hated me.

My next thought was that I could design a massage tool that would be easier on my hands.

There was an inherent problem with this idea, which is that I'm pretty good at destroying things, but not so good at building things. (Just ask my wife, Lisa.)

Fortunately, my dad—a Depression era kid who could build a house with toothpicks, old newspapers and discarded dental floss—was up for the job and together we created a lot of massage tools, like "the monster tool."

The monster tool is aptly named. The tip of the monster tool (pictured below) was over 2 inches long and looked like a drill bit.

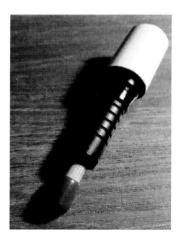

(P3)

The handle was about 14 inches long, and the butt of the handle would rest in the front of my armpit.

The monster tool soon became my favorite tool, but no client ever saw it. Can you imagine being on the massage table and seeing what looked like a drill bit coming at your forearm?

Over the next ten years I brought all my Dad-made massage tools into the massage room with me, but to my dismay none of the tools, including my beloved monster tool, saved my hands.

As my business grew, my body started racking up more damage, like the cervical radiculopathy, cubital tunnel syndrome, and unstable left shoulder that I mentioned in the opening.

The Massage Pain-Free Experiment

In one last attempt to save my massage career, I gave myself an ultimatum: You have a year to fix your body or you quit massage.

The good news was that I wasn't starting from scratch. I knew that there was no perfect tool that was going to solve my hand pain issue, and I also learned that using a variety of massage tools reduced some hand pain because I wasn't stressing the same muscles in my hands all the time.

The question was, why didn't using a variety of massage tools stop my hand pain altogether?

The answer had literally been staring me in the face for years, and the monster tool held the key.

Though the monster tool looked like it should be part of a dawn-of-dentistry tool kit, it had one advantage over all the other tools. It was designed so that the handle fit into the front of an armpit. To exert pressure you pinned the monster tool between the front of your armpit and the tissue you were working on and then leaned. You could then relax your holding-hand because you only needed to steady the massage tool since your body weight was doing all the work.

So, what if I took the monster tool "pin and lean" concept and applied it to all massage tool usage? It was my "it's not the dog, it's the dog owner" revelation. The *tool* wasn't the problem, it was how I was *holding* the tool.

Instead of using the NMT "grip the tip" approach to holding the T-bar, I tried the monster tool "pin and lean" idea to hold the T-bar and sure enough, I was able to relax my grip. In fact, I could even open my hand.

As I experimented with the pin and lean technique I soon discovered that I could steady the massage tool in many different ways. I was like a kid in a candy store as I explored the different holds.

I have to admit that at the same time I was experiencing this breakthrough joy, I also sort of wanted to cry. The joy part was that I'd essentially figured out how to save my hands. The crying part was, "Seriously, dude? It took you this long to figure that out?"

But I wasn't out of the woods yet—my shoulder, elbow and neck still hurt. Fixing my other body parts required some introspection, which wasn't as straightforward as pinning and leaning with a massage tool. Here's the insight that proved to be key: I'm a smiley-face collector. I want to please people. If I make someone happy, I get a shot of dopamine—boom!—and life is good.

It's not surprising that I chose a career where I can get shots of dopamine all day long. When a client gets off my table, she's happy (most of the time), and that means Mark is not only going to get paid, he's also going to get a shot of dopamine. Sweet. And this goes on all day long. What other job gives you that many opportunities for collecting smiley faces? Not a lot.

I'm thinking that being a people-pleaser is probably one of the reasons you do massage too, and that your internal pharmacist is also cranking out the dopamine.

But here's a potential problem: If you're like me, all that people-pleasing dopamine can override the pain tolerance or self-preservation mechanism. In other words, we get the dopamine reward for jamming our thumb into Toral's lamina groove to help her back pain go away, but we also get a thumb that hurts more and more with each deep tissue massage we do, which is a set up for a major showdown between their pain versus my pain.

Their Pain Versus My Pain

I remember a "their pain versus my pain" showdown that had a major impact on how I do massage to this day. Alex was my last massage of a long day. I was a month or so into my year-long experiment to eliminate pain when doing massage, and though I had been experimenting with different ways to hold massage tools, my fingers were still a little cranky.

I was about to do supine work on Alex's tight neck, and I could feel myself tensing as I anticipated the pain that was about to occur in my hands when a voice in my head said: "Why are you doing supine neck work when you know it hurts your fingers?"

The question stunned and exhilarated me at the same time. The stunning part was that the question revealed that I hadn't *really* been looking out for my body because I was continuing to do techniques that hurt my body. The exhilarating part was that I finally recognized that this was a *choice*.

So I picked up a T-bar with a thin stem.

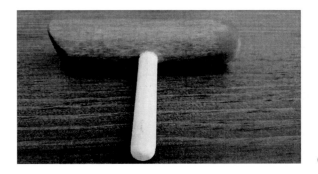

(P4)

And with a guide finger down next to the tip I started with prone neck work. When I felt that I was losing sensitivity I switched to a thumb, and when that thumb started to feel a little discomfort I switched to two thumbs bracing each other. I went back and forth between massage tool, thumb and barred thumbs without ever working on Alex's neck in the supine position. And at the end of the massage, my fingers felt good.

The horse was out of the barn—forever. Now I could pick and choose which technique to use with each client. If I wanted to save my fingers for a client I knew only wanted supine neck work, I could—by using other neck techniques on clients I knew didn't have a preference.

If you're thinking "yay, massage pain-free", but "boo, massage tools", don't worry, you don't have to use massage tools to massage pain-free.

Using massage tools is only one strategy to massage pain-free. There are many more, which I explain in this book.

Some of the strategies may seem straightforward, like "become ambidextrous", and some, like "short stroke massage", may seem weird. But I promise you that by the end of this book, all the strategies and techniques I show you will make sense.

By the way, you don't have to master all the strategies to massage pain-free. Take in these strategies the way Bruce Lee, the famous martial artist, approached new information: "Research your own experience. Absorb what is useful, reject what is useless, add what is essentially your own".[1]

That said, this book is about strategies, not axioms. Work a strategy. If it's a fit for your body, problem solved. If not, modify it or move on to the next one. My goal is not to be your trail blazer. My goal is to give you the tools so that you can blaze your own trail to massaging pain-free.

Lastly, I know you're worried about losing clients if you change the way you massage—I was. The reality is that initially you may lose a few, but think about what you'll ultimately gain—a way to do massage that doesn't hurt you, more clients over time, and more years in a career that you love.

To set yourself up for a long career in massage, it may look like I'm asking you to break some time-honored rules. Well, if one of those rules is causing you pain when you massage, then I'm guilty as charged. There's a good reason for that and it's not because I'm a contrarian. In fact, I have a great deal of respect for the rule-makers. It's simply because if I *hadn't* broken some of the rules, my massage career would have ended a long time ago.

But as you can see, I'm still here, known as a therapist with the ability to deliver deep pressure, closing in on thirty years with plenty left in the tank. And that is what I want for you.

Introduction:
Put Your Own Mask on First

What are you doing when the flight attendant starts to explain the emergency procedures for plane evacuation? I'm usually trying to send one last text or email on my phone before it has to be shut off or put on airplane mode. But I know that even though I've heard the safety spiel a thousand times, I *should* still pay attention because this could be the time I actually need it.

Imagine you're flying over the Atlantic Ocean, above the clouds, and suddenly the plane dips. Over the loud speaker the pilot instructs the flight staff to prepare the passengers for an emergency landing. Your mom sitting next to you is panicking, fumbling for her mask, and is now struggling to breathe.

We all know the famous line in the flight attendant's mask message—*put your own mask on first*—so that you don't run out of air, because you can't help the person next to you if you're dead. Would you actually follow the directive you'd so often tuned out?

Now imagine that every time the flight attendant gave the safety spiel you not only listened, you actually pictured yourself putting on your own mask first before helping the person next to you. You also thought about the rationale for doing this. Do your chances for following the directive go up because you've reinforced that directive in your mind?

I'm thinking yes.

Now let's apply this analogy to a massage day. Remember a time in the massage room when your thumb ached, or your back tightened up, or your traps screamed at you, or your head was too heavy for your neck.

What did you do?

Did you put on your own oxygen mask on first?

Did you take care of your pain before you took care of your client's pain?

I can't help but think of my wife, Lisa, at this moment. She's a massage therapist with fibromyalgia who works through a lot of physical pain. Yet, she will tolerate more pain on top of a baseline of pain to get the job done, because her instinct is to help someone else first and to think about her pain second.

It's hard to short circuit that instinct because there's no flight attendant telling you to put your own oxygen mask on first.

That is, until now. I'll be the flight attendant.

Think about your own pain first.

One more time: *Think about your own pain first.*

Once more: *Think about your own pain first.*

Now you take over as the flight attendant. Say it: *Think about my own pain first.*

Next, let's create the "think about my own pain first" loop that needs to be running in your brain at all times. To facilitate this we're going to make this pain personal.

Pick an area on your body that talks to you when you're on massage number four of the day.

Mine was T3, in between my spine and scapula, on the left side.

Imagine you start to feel your pain during a massage. For me, I'm imagining that I'm working on Taro's tight lower back and that T3 hot poker is about to send nerve tingling down my arm.

What do you normally do? You work through it, right? Why? Because working through pain is what you do. It's a habit, until you can't work through the pain, and then you do less massage or quit doing massage altogether.

But this time instead of working through the pain, I'm going to have you interrupt that habit by asking yourself this question: How do I get the job done without being in pain? How do I get the job done on Taro's back without a hot poker?

First, I take a second to break from the static posture that I've been in for 5 minutes by switching to one-handed massage so that I can straighten up my back. That immediately relieves some of the pain in my upper-back.

Then I remember that when I use my forearm to work Taro's lower back I often feel that hot poker. So, I stop using my forearm and switch to knuckles. That really helps my hot poker area, but now I can't generate enough pressure because I didn't set my table low enough since I wasn't anticipating that I'd be using my knuckles on Taro's lower back.

Don't give up, Mark, keep thinking.

Aha! Where Taro really likes deep pressure is around L5. I'll have him turn on his side and I can do some focus work in that area with my knuckles in a seated leaning position. I know that working on someone in the side posture does not aggravate my hot poker spot.

You can start to see that by asking the question—how do I get the job done without being in pain?—you get creative. And when you get creative, you find ways to save your body without compromising your work.

By the way, you may have noticed that in the Taro example I wasn't actually prepared to work on Taro in a way that wouldn't cause me pain.

I was thinking on the fly. Thinking on the fly is important to massaging pain-free, but it's only half of the equation. Setting yourself up for success is the other half. Together, setting yourself up for success and thinking on the fly equal the best solution for massaging pain-free.

How do you set yourself up for success to massage pain-free?

You ask yourself—How do I massage without being in pain?—before the massage even starts.

If I had asked myself that question before Taro got on the table, I would have lowered my table so that I could get enough leaning leverage to work Taro's lower-back with my knuckles and fists.

I also would have brought a massage tool, like a T-bar, into the massage room with me for focus work in Taro's lower-back. The T-bar would not only give my knuckles a break, it would also allow me to easily generate focused pressure.

It seems pretty straight forward so far, right?

Our automatic pilot is set to work through pain. To short circuit the automatic pilot or to interrupt the habit of working through pain, you have to ask yourself, "How do I massage without being in pain?"—before the massage and during the massage.

But it's not quite that simple. There are a lot of reasons why a habit develops and some of the reasons may not show up on your normal, waking-state radar. So, let's be sure that you can recognize when and why you might be working through pain.

Kate is a part-time massage therapist who worked for us while she had a full-time, non-massage job. Before she worked for us, she had stopped massage entirely because of shoulder pain. Her shoulder didn't bother her the first year that she worked for us, but she was starting to feel it in year two.

So Kate and I went into the massage room to see what we could figure out. I was the body on the table (oh, the sacrifices I make to help others) and Kate started to work on me, but for the longest time Kate couldn't reproduce the shoulder pain that threatened to sideline her again.

That was my first clue that Kate was not attentive to her body during the massage. Eventually, she reproduced the pain doing a subscapularis technique on me.

Okay, we had something to work with now. As Kate continued to perform the subscap technique on me, her confidence grew that this move was the singular culprit behind her shoulder pain.

So I suggested an alternative subscap technique to her.

Kate tried it, and the move didn't cause her any shoulder pain.

Fantastic! I was ready to collect the smiley faces due to me, but to my surprise Kate stiffed me.

In fact, Kate looked upset. So I sucked up my indignation and asked her what was up.

She said, "I can't believe that I didn't think about trying a different move."

Now, I need to explain that Kate was also a researcher. Obviously, she was used to analyzing and figuring things out, and she was embarrassed and disappointed that she hadn't figured out how to solve her pain issue herself.

But as Kate and I talked, it became clear that there was an emotional barrier preventing her from solving her pain issue. You see, the subscap technique that hurt Kate's shoulder was her signature move. She loved doing that move and, in her mind, it defined her as a massage therapist.

Was she really going to give up that move and be like every other massage therapist around her?

I get it. It took me months to accept that certain techniques— techniques that my clients loved—hurt my body. And to be honest, I didn't really accept it. With great hesitancy I inserted experimental moves for the moves that hurt me and I watched, like a hawk, for negative reactions from my clients.

At the end of the day, with some more experimenting and tweaking, my clients usually liked my substitute moves as much as they did my original moves. And guess what? My substitute moves—that didn't hurt my body—were now my signature moves that defined me as a massage therapist.

I know I'm asking a lot. I'm asking you to put your own mask on first by asking yourself, "How do I get the job done without being in pain?"—before and during each massage.

Then I'm asking you to be open to experimentation, knowing that you may have to jettison techniques that hurt your body—some that may be signature techniques—and replace them with ones that don't.

And then the big ask: Trust my experience. My experience showed me that new techniques that didn't hurt my body could replace old techniques that did hurt my body (even signature moves) AND I would not lose my sense of self as a massage therapist.

That's a lot, I know, but I promise you that there are big rewards waiting at the other end.

Lastly, this book is divided into two parts. Part One is a general strategy for eliminating neck, shoulder, arm and back pain.

The strategy is to lean to generate pressure. The premise is that when you use your body weight to generate pressure, you take your upper-body out of the strain equation.

I was amazed, and I think you will be too, how many neck, shoulder, arm and back pain issues simply disappear when the upper-body doesn't have to be taxed during a massage.

In Part Two, Taking Pain-Free to the Next Level, you will experiment with specific strategies and techniques to eliminate neck, back, shoulder, arm, wrist and hand pain. Also, if you go to www.painfreemassagetherapist.com there are free, instructional videos to help make things stick.

The first thing we're going to do is to break some unconscious rules and challenge the entrenched and non-useful ways of thinking that are preventing you from massaging pain-free.

Part 1

THE FOUNDATION FOR PAIN-FREE MASSAGE

CHAPTER ONE

Lean

I was first introduced to the strategy of leaning to generate pressure by a massage therapist named Xentho, aka, "X."

One day X showed up at my office door in a fitness center, looking for a job. He was nice and easy to talk to, but there was no getting around the fact that he was a 250 lb. rugby player who could crush me like a grape. How were clients going to react to his physical stature?

Well, he had an answer for that. "Let me work on you," he said.

With some reservation I agreed to get on the table, and to my surprise, X didn't break me. In fact, he had great hands and his pressure was spot on from my calves to neck. I hired him right then and clients loved him.

Over the next year, X and I became friends and once when we were chatting in the office he gave it to me straight.

He said, "Mark, you're always hurt and you got all those tools and everything, but you're not doing it right. You're working too hard."

Okay, I said, thinking that what works for you, X, is that you're 250 lbs. of muscle. Lend me about 75 lbs. of muscle and I'll be good too.

Nevertheless, I went out on the workout floor and grabbed my personal trainer friend, John, who loved massage and would give me honest feedback.

After John was on the table, X and I entered the room. X started to work on John's back and that's when I really started to pay attention. X wasn't muscling through the massage the way I thought he was going to, and the way I did at the time. In fact, it looked like he was barely exerting any effort at all.

What was X doing?

He was transferring his body weight onto John with his forearm as the contact point. In other words, he was just leaning on John.

"This is how you do it," he said to me.

How does it feel? I asked John.

"Oh, my God," said John, "it feels like more."

I looked back at X and he smiled then closed his eyes, pretending he was sleeping as he massaged.

John continued to groan his approval.

"Pull up an elbow," X said to me.

On the other side of John's back I tried to mimic what X was doing, and X gave me feedback.

"You're working too hard."

"Rest."

"Close your eyes."

"Go to sleep."

Sleep?

Massage is work, I said.

X shook his head disapprovingly.

After a while I was getting frustrated because every time I looked at X he was so chill, which was in direct contrast to how I felt as I struggled to relax into the massage. But then John gave me some encouragement.

"That's good," he said, "it feels like the pressure X is using."

Hmm...I checked in with my body.

Shoulders relaxed? Check. Back relaxed? Yep. How about hands? Now they are. Hey! I'm relaxed and my body weight is doing all the work!

I looked over at X to express my approval. His eyes were still closed and this time I swear he was really asleep.

Wake up, I said.

Without opening his eyes he chuckled and then said, "Not dreaming yet."

I wish that I could say from that point on I mastered X's leaning and was pain-free in the massage room, but I'd be lying.

The truth is that I understood only the immediate application of using my body weight to generate force with my forearm while doing back work. That's all.

I didn't get the *universal* application of leaning until 10-ish years later when my massage body was in the final stage of falling apart.

That's when, out of sheer survival, I learned that leaning—transferring my body weight onto the client—could reduce muscular tension in my neck, shoulders, arms and back no matter the pressure (light to deep), no matter the type of work (focused to relaxation), and no matter the body type (small to large).

How?

It's simple. My body weight is doing the work when I lean. The only thing I need to do is direct and stabilize my body weight. That doesn't take much work.

So, no more crazy pressing with my shoulders and arms. Neck muscles now can relax. Shoulders, elbows and wrists are protected because they are in alignment. And I can even straighten my back while I'm working.

But there was a sticky wicket to being able to lean anywhere, anytime—and that was table height.

When X taught me how to lean and use my forearm on a client's back I stopped straining my upper-body, but, over time, because of my specific injury, the pressure from leaning with my forearm fired up my T3 area. I needed another body part to use that was like a forearm, but impacted my shoulder less. I didn't have to look too far down my arm to find a substitute. Hello, fists.

But wait, if I were leaning on the client with my fists I would need more distance between me and the client than I would if I were leaning on the client with my forearm.

To illustrate this, stand behind the back of a couch or imagine you're standing behind the back of a couch. Now bend your arm and lean on the back of the couch with your fore-arm. Depending on the height of the back of the couch you can probably generate a fair amount of pressure by letting the couch support your body weight.

Now try it with your fists, keeping your arms straight. Not working so well, right? There's not enough distance between your fists and the back of the couch for you to transfer your body weight onto the back of the couch.

Walk around to the arms of the couch which are lower than the back of the couch. Now lean with your fists into the armrests so that you're almost doing a plank on your fists. Transferring your body weight is no problem, right?

So, the proper table height for leaning is low?

Unfortunately, the answer is not that straight-forward. The right table height for you to lean effectively and without being in pain will depend on (1) your specific chronic conditions and/or new injuries, (2) massage styles (if you use parallel foot stances in addition to asymmetrical foot stances), and (3) certain on-the-spot considerations, like client size.

I know leaning is starting to sound complicated, but if we examine these points we can arrive at some general conclusions and that will make deciding on table height easier for you. I'm going to use myself as an example.

Chronic Conditions and New Injuries

As I mentioned previously, my friend X introduced me to leaning with my forearm/elbow. Over time, leaning with my forearm/elbow, exacerbated my shoulder and neck conditions enough so that I didn't want to lean with my forearm/elbow any longer.

So that meant I needed to switch my massage style. Eventually, during my year-long experiment to save my body, I switched to fists and I figured out that a low table when using my fists was the optimal setting for allowing me to leverage my body weight onto a client.

Not all chronic conditions and new injuries will have such a dramatic impact on how you lean, but you should be aware that some could. For me, I switched from doing 60% of a massage with an elbow/forearm to 60% massage with fists. Since it was a chronic condition I needed a long-term fix and not a short-term one.

Here's an example of a short-term fix for an injury that was going to go away. A while back I borrowed my brother-in-law's truck and closed the tailgate too hard which resulted in a jammed middle finger on my right hand. It was a bad jam and there was no way I was using that finger during a massage.

To substitute for that finger I used a T-bar with a long stem that extended past the length of my middle finger. At the time, my table was too high to use the T-bar effectively. So, I lowered my table for the next 3 weeks while my finger healed.

Do you always need to lower your table to adjust to a pain condition or injury?

No. It will depend on your style and your injury. Once, I tweaked my upper back when working out and I raised my table up two notches until the injury healed.

In general, chronic pain issues will influence your table height selection every day. Acute injuries and conditions will influence your table height selection for brief periods of time.

Before we talk about the next criteria for selecting a table height—asymmetrical versus parallel foot stances—we need to talk about body mechanics as it relates to leaning.

The Body Mechanics Study That Helped Me

Towards the end of my year-long experiment I came across an interesting body mechanics study. Edward Mohr, massage therapist and once ergonomics engineering manager, ran a computer modeling test and conducted a field study to evaluate the best body mechanics for producing maximal force. His study was published in the Journal of Bodywork and Movement Therapies in 2010.[2]

He concluded that good posture, which included leaning, stacking joints and locking a leg when in an asymmetrical stance, "correlated with an overall 34% increase in applied maximal force, as compared with the improper posture."[3]

In essence, Mohr's study validated my experience that leaning was king for generating force efficiently and safely.

Mohr writes: "The other key principle in massage is that body weight and gravity are free. Making movements in a downward direction, the weight of the body can be used to increase the force (Konz, 1995). Normally, whenever the center of gravity of the body moves past the base of the feet, some muscles contract to counteract and stabilize the body. However, when that force generated by body weight can be transferred through the hand onto another stationary object, this force transfer requires only minimal muscle activity. Also, since the majority of the force is generated through body weight, the force can be applied for a longer time period without generating undue fatigue."[4]

To this day, I'm still amazed at how I'm barely working when I'm leaning.

On my blog, www.makethemostofmassage.com, I wrote posts describing leaning as "minimal effort massage". Lisa said that sounded like "lazy massage". Then I came up with "maximal efficiency massage". That got me, "You mean 'more important sounding than it is' massage?" For now, I'm sticking with just "leaning" and letting the experience of leaning speak for itself.

In addition to validating my experience of leaning as an efficient way to generate pressure, Mohr's study provided two other findings that make for a happy body when leaning to generate force. The first one is stacking joints.

Stacking Joints

In the study, Mohr explains that joints have to counteract the rotational effects of moments on them. A moment is a rotational movement around an axis. Stacking arm joints minimizes the rotational effects of moments at those joints.[5]

This explanation probably doesn't wow you at this point because you haven't experienced how easy it is to stabilize your body weight when your arm joints are stacked. So, let's get on that.

Stacking

What are we stacking?

Shoulders, elbows and wrists.

Here I'm stacking while I'm using my fists:

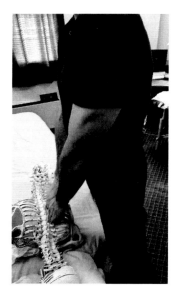

(1.1)

22

And here I'm stacking my shoulder over my elbow while using my forearm:

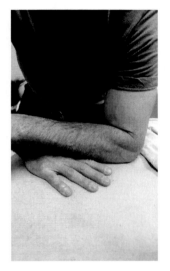

(1.2)

Imagine if I moved my elbow about 3 inches in, where my belt buckle is, while keeping my shoulder in the same place as it is in the picture, and then leaned with all of my weight.

That alignment should make you cringe, especially if you imagine me doing a plank in this position.

Give me a plank with elbow 3 inches away from your shoulder and hold those planks for 60 seconds!

That's something you're never going to hear a personal trainer say because she knows it could stress your shoulder joint and lead to a shoulder injury. Stacking makes stabilizing your body weight easy.

The other finding in Mohr's study that made for a "happy body while leaning" was locking.

Locking

Specifically, Mohr is talking about locking the back knee in an asymmetrical stance (lunge stance). When your leg is locked you can drive (push) from the locked leg to generate additional force.

In the picture below I'm in an asymmetrical stance.

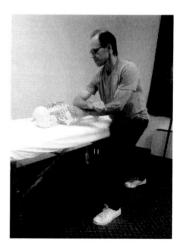

(1.3)

My back knee is locked and my front leg is bent. If I wanted to ramp up my pressure, I would push from my back leg.

Locking the back knee when in an asymmetrical stance, like a lunge stance, and driving from the heel of that leg is a key ingredient to delivering more force in Mohr's study.

My experience in the massage room and Mohr's study seemed like a marriage made in heaven.

Lean. Check.

Stack joints. Check.

Lock the back leg when in an asymmetrical stance to generate more power. Check.

But then the bad news—there was an inference that could be made from the study that didn't jibe with my massage room experience. The inference from Mohr's study is this: A higher table is better than a lower table when leaning to apply pressure.

Let me explain how someone might come to this determination even though it is not stated as a conclusion in the study.

In the field study, Mohr set out to test maximal force with 5 different postures. He wanted to see if proper posture (stacked, locked and leaning) beat out improper posture (arm push with no-to-little leaning) in terms of maximal force at three application heights.

He chose 29 inches, 34.5 inches and 39.5 inches for his application heights and had massage therapists press against the edge of a simulated massage table at these 3 different heights. Using an Ergo-FET digital palm force gauge he was able to record maximal force readings at each application with each posture.

He found "that proper body mechanics correlated with an overall 34% increase in applied maximal force, as compared with the improper posture".[6] Another way of saying that is that the massage therapist was able to deliver more force using proper body mechanics at all the application heights than she could when she was using improper body mechanics.

He also concluded, "the impact of using proper body mechanics being greatest at the highest point of application."[7]

So, the biggest "maximal force" bang for the buck happened at 39.5 inches. This is where the inference comes in that it's better to work on a high table than a low table, because you can generate more force on a high table.

This wasn't adding up for me. My experience said that I could apply plenty of force, effortlessly, on a *low* table.

It took me some time and a discussion with Mohr himself to understand that this inference was inaccurate, and it had to do with the limitations of the study.

The most significant limitation in the study was application heights (the table height at which the subject's hands applied pressure to the edge of a simulated massage table). As I mentioned before, Mohr used three application heights in the study: 39.5, 34.5 and 29 inches.

The highest setting for my massage table, measuring from floor to the top of the table, is 33.5 inches. That means two of the application heights in the study are out of the range of the absolute highest setting on my table. Also, 29 inches was the lowest application height in the study.

Guess what my table height is set at?

Twenty-two and half inches. That's 6.5 inches lower than the lowest application height in the study. So, there *was* no maximal force test at a *truly* low application height in the study. Even if there *had* been a truly low application height in the study, in order to fairly assess maximal force on a low table, the experimenter would have to test the best body mechanics postures *for* a low table, which, in my experience, are not entirely the same as best body mechanics postures for a high table. In my view, using only the best body mechanics postures for a high table inadvertently biased the study against low tables.

I agree with Mohr that stacking joints and locking the back leg when in an asymmetrical stance are key for generating force efficiently at most table heights, but unlike a high table, a low table opens the door for a parallel foot stance.

If you watch me massage you would see that I'm often over-top the client, like a chiropractor or a shiatsu practitioner. A parallel foot stance makes it easy to get to muscles closer to the midline of the person on the table. It's my go-to stance when I'm applying focused pressure with double knuckles or massage tools in the thoracic and lumbar lamina groove.

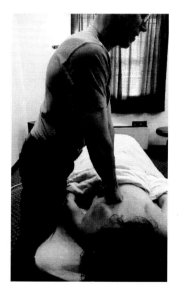

(1.4)

You may be wondering how I apply pressure in a parallel foot stance when there is no back leg to lock and push from to generate additional force like I do when I'm in the asymmetrical stance.

The answer?

Body weight.

With a low table I am able to leverage most of my body weight onto the client if I need to. With a high table in an asymmetrical stance, I can only leverage some body weight—the rest of the pressure has to be generated through leg power.

Mohr is not a fan of low tables or the parallel foot stance.

In an AMTA video where he's demonstrating Sandy Fritz's (massage therapist, author and educator) body-mechanics principles, he points out that in the parallel-foot stance the massage therapist's back is doing some major work during the transition phase from standing to leaning into the client.[8]

His point is spot on and I've experienced back discomfort firsthand. But there's a remedy for this: Don't let your back hang out in la-la land, the transition zone between standing and leaning into the client/table. In other words, get from point A, standing, to point B, where your body weight is supported by the client and/or table, without hesitation so that you don't stress your back.

Mohr also points out in the video that the parallel foot stance could strain your back when doing light to medium pressure.[9]

Again, he's spot on.

If you're in the parallel foot stance when doing deep pressure you're okay because you're transferring most of your weight onto the client so your back doesn't have to do a lot of work to support your body. But if the client wants lighter pressure, then you have to shift some of your weight to your heels. Now your back is working to support your body weight again.

Here's how you solve the challenge with light to medium pressure when in the parallel foot stance: First, make sure that the fronts of your legs are actually leaning into the table. This will help support your body weight.

Next, step back from the table a little and widen your stance. Now you can lean more of your body weight into the table and the wider stance will allow you to straighten up so that you can put your back in a neutral position. Those two adjustments will take the strain out of your back.

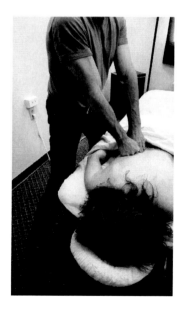

(1.5)

Another solution is to put a knee on the table in a way that doesn't touch the client or make the client uncomfortable, like on the edge of the table. This position puts you directly over your client with most of your body weight supported by the table.

In the next chapter I'll go into more detail about how to use the massage table to help support your body. By the way, these support-your-body-using-a massage-table techniques can be used at any table height setting.

If it sounds like I'm planting a flag on the parallel-foot-stance/ low table hill, I'm not.

And there's no disrespect meant towards Sandy Fritz or Edward Mohr. In fact, thank you Sandy Fritz and Edward Mohr for your vitally important work which helped me complete my body mechanics toolkit.

I'm advocating for the parallel foot stance and/or a low table if they prove to work with *your* massage style and body givens, including chronic conditions. Period. The question each massage therapist should be asking is not, "which is the right table height, low or high?". It's, "which is the right table height for *me*?". Don't let anyone, including me, answer that question for you.

Now, let's take a look at four on-the-spot considerations that will help you decide how high or low you set your table.

On-The-Spot Considerations

The on-the-spot considerations are the: (1) primary body part you're using to deliver pressure, (2) size of the client, (3) primary area of focus (e.g. low back or glutes), (4) and pressure the client wants.

You will get this information before the client gets onto your table through your intake process. Once you have this information, you can set your table height accordingly.

Let's look at the first on-the-spot consideration for setting the height of your massage table:

1. The primary body part you're using to deliver pressure.

We already touched on that with the couch example, but let's put some flesh on the bones.

Auria is a client of mine who loves super-deep pressure. Before my injuries, I'd mainly use forearms on Auria. I'd set my table height three holes from the bottom. At this height I had enough distance between her back and my forearm so I could lean all my body weight into her.

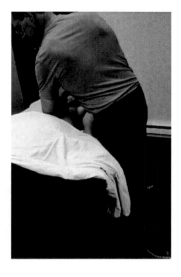

(1.6)

When I switched to fists and tried to transfer all my body weight into Auria on a table set for forearms, it didn't work.

Why?

Just like in the couch example, there wasn't enough distance between me and Auria for me to lean all my body weight into her.

Eventually, I dropped my table to the lowest setting and, lo and behold, I had enough distance to lean into her back with all of my body weight using my fists as the contact points with her body.

In general, fists, knuckles, fingers, palms and massage tools require more leaning distance than forearms.

What about the size of a client? Does that make a difference in how you set your table height? It sure does.

2. The size of the client.

David, who weighs 305 lbs, is "thicker" than Abdul Hai who weighs 150. That means if David and Abdul Hai were lying on a table side-by-side, the top of David's body would be an inch or two higher off the table than Abdul Hai's.

If you set your table height at the Abdul Hai level for each massage, you'd be giving up an inch or two of leaning leverage when working on someone big, like David. We all know what happens when you can't lean to generate pressure. You have to press like a maniac with your upper body, and then your body hates you, then you hate massage, and you look for a book like this one. Let's not start that cycle again.

The next consideration when choosing a table height is the primary area of focus for the massage: where you'll be doing most of your work. Are you going to be spending most of your time on a hill or in a valley?

3. Primary Area of Focus – Hills Versus Valleys

Imagine Carol is lying prone on your massage table. Her glutes will stick up off the table higher than her calves, right? Glutes are hills. Calves are valleys. When looking at the back, the thoracic back is a hill and the lumbar back is a valley.

Say Carol is a "body parts" massage and she wants deep focus work on her glutes, a hill in our analogy. You use your fists as your primary body part to apply pressure and you use both asymmetrical and parallel foot stances.

At your normal low table height, you can lean into Carol's legs, a valley, using your fists with deep pressure—no problem. But to be able to lean to generate deep pressure into her glutes, a hill, you'd have to get on your tiptoes.

What's the solution to have leaning leverage for Carol glutes?

Set the table height for Carol's glutes, not her calves, which means you'll need a lower table than your normal table height.

Now imagine Carol wants you to work on her lumbar back, a valley. You're a forearm massager and stick to asymmetrical stances, which means you generate additional force by driving from your back leg.

You typically set your table for Carol's thoracic back, a hill, because that is where she wants her focus work, but this time Carol requests her lower back, a valley. In this case, setting your table for Carol's lumbar back may require you to raise your table.

To keep it simple, valleys may require a higher-than-normal table and hills may require a lower-than-normal table.

Don't over-think this. It will all make sense once you start practicing.

The last on-the-spot consideration we need to talk about is the pressure the client wants.

4. The pressure the client wants.

Light pressure is less important in terms of dialing in on table height because if you're working on a high table your back will not be in flexion and if you're working on a low table you can use the massage table to support your body weight.

However, a request for medium or deep pressure should make your ears prick up because you'll need to generate more force. If you want to use more body weight than leg power, then you'll lower your table to lean.

At this point, you may have noticed that I've given you a lot of information regarding setting your table height, but I haven't given you an exact table height setting to try. There's a good reason: I don't know what your exact setting should be.

My arms may be longer or shorter than yours. My injuries and pain issues may or may not be the same as yours. I may or may not have more deep pressure clients. And I may or may not have more body parts clients than you do. So, you'll need to experiment to figure out your table height.

That said, I have two starting table height recommendations for your experiment—one notch higher than your normal table height and at least one, but no more than 3 notches lower than your normal table height.

That's not to say that you can't settle on a table height more than 3 notches below your normal table height or more than 1 notch above your normal table height. I'm just giving you a guide that will ease your way into both high and low table leaning.

Why two recommendations?

I gave you two so that you can experiment with high table leaning and low table leaning and then compare those to leaning at your normal table height.

Before you experiment with leaning, especially with a lower table, promise me you'll finish this chapter and the next one. Let's just say leaning can get ugly fast, especially low table leaning, if you don't know how to use the table to support your body weight. By the way, in addition to supporting your body weight, the massage table can also help you regulate pressure.

Years ago, Joe, a massage therapist I was teaching, helped me really understand the table-as-a–regulator-of-pressure concept.

Joe wouldn't lean. I tried everything. I almost jumped on his back. His sticking point was that he was afraid that he was going to hurt the person on the table.

Finally one day, I broke Joe (in a good way). It went something like this: Rick, another MT, was on the table and Joe was using his forearms on Ricks' back.

I asked Rick how the pressure was.

"Light."

Joe repositioned himself and leaned some more.

How about now?, I asked.

"Still the same."

This went on another 3 or 4 times. It baffled me because on each try, Joe repositioned himself and then applied pressure. It looked like he was really bringing it.

What was going on here?

I looked closer at Joe's body position and that's when I found out that he was tricking us good. He wasn't leaning most of his body weight into Rick. He was leaning primarily into the table.

Poor Joe, that's when I tortured his soul.

No more legs leaning into the table. I made Joe plank on Rick. Okay, I didn't make him plank, but I did make him lean until he was at the pressure where Rick said, "Perfect."

Getting someone on the table to say "the pressure is perfect" as you learn how to use your body weight to apply pressure will take some practice, but stick with it—even when it feels wrong. That feeling of "wrong" is just that, a feeling. It happens because you haven't given yourself enough time to let an alternative to muscling your way through a massage to settle in. The best alternative to muscling your way through a massage is leaning. And the best way to feel like leaning is normal is to get reps in.

When you're getting your reps in make sure the person on the table can give you good feedback, likes deep pressure and is okay to receive deep pressure.

Leaning with all your body weight will feel weird at first because we all have some Joe in us. What I mean is none of us want to hurt a client by using too much pressure.

You're not going to hurt clients or yourself because in the next chapter I'm going to talk about how to use the table to regulate pressure and support your body.

Though this section was developed specifically for low table leaning, it can be applied to leaning at all table heights. Remember, your choice as to whether you're a high-, medium- or low-table leaner will ultimately depend on what feels best to your body and works with your massage style.

Before we move into using the table for support and to regulate pressure, I want to say this: I'm lazy. I don't want to think that much about adjusting my table height for each massage. So, to make sure that I'm always prepared for deep pressure, I set my table height as low as possible (with the lower table legs off) at 22.5 inches.

That said, I'm 5' 11", at least I was yesterday. A therapist at 5'3" who is a low-table leaner will want a lower table than mine. Good news; some big brands make tables that go as low as 17.5 inches. Sometimes these tables are listed as medi-sport therapy or treatment tables. You can find a list of massage tables that go lower than standard tables at www.painfreemassagetherapist.com.

Lastly, working on a low table presents a couple of body mechanics challenges, but I'm going to show you the work-arounds in the next chapter.

CHAPTER TWO

Use the Table for Support and to Regulate Pressure

Finally, I get to talk about my best friend—my massage table (as far as inanimate objects are concerned).

There's a good reason why my massage table is my best inanimate-object friend. When I was doing my year-long experiment to save my body, it saved my back.

Let me backtrack for a minute. I had three rules that I followed in my year-long experiment:

1. Figure out what triggered or caused me pain in the massage room.

2. Stop doing the things that triggered/caused pain.

3. Find alternatives to get the job done.

The first problem area on my body that I addressed was my T3 hot-poker.

A trigger for my T3 hot-poker was leaning with my forearm.

So, I stopped leaning with my forearm and started leaning with my fists.

The result was that my T3 hot-poker pain went away, but now I had lumbar pain from working on a very low table when doing light to medium pressure clients.

You probably noticed that I didn't say deep pressure bothered my back when working on a low table.

You already know the reason why. I could lean all my body weight into a deep pressure client and that meant less work for my postural muscles. But with light to medium I had to control how much of my body weight was going into the client which meant more work for my back.

I was in denial about the back pain from working on a low table with light to medium clients because my T3 area was feeling so good, but one day it was just too much. To give myself a rest I put a leg against the table.

There was a twofold reward when I did this. First, using the table to help support my body weight took the strain out of my back.

The other reward was that it made light and medium pressure easy to do because I didn't have to work hard to stay upright since the table was now supporting the body weight that wasn't being directed into the client. In fact, it allowed me to regulate my leaning pressure with surgical precision.

Lean Into the Table to Support Your Back

When you put a leg against your table, your world is going to change because your postural muscles will be doing less work to keep you upright.

The key to leaning against the table is to **actually put a leg (or two) against the table so that you can experiment.**

This requires some attention to where your leg is contacting the table. Obviously, you don't want your leg touching the client. You're looking for a clean edge on the table with no client body parts in the way. Sometimes I move the client's arm on or off the table to get a clean edge for my leg.

At first this may seem awkward, as in *I should be massaging instead of looking for a place to put my leg.* But once you start reaping the rewards of a leg against the table, that thought will evaporate and you'll instinctively find the clean edge of the table for your leg all the time.

There's no one way to lean into the table. In fact, you can lean into the massage table for support with all sides of your legs—front, back, side, and inside. And it doesn't take a lot of your weight directed into the table for you to feel your back being supported.

When I lean into the table with one leg, I make contact with the table just above my knee cap. Where you contact the table with your leg may be different. Remember this is a

DIY book where you're figuring out what works for you, not what works for me. In the picture below most of my weight is going into the client and the table is providing me with some extra support for my back.

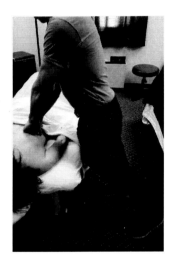

(2.1)

What about leaning with two legs? That may seem odd at first, but here's a scenario where two legs against the table is key to supporting your back and regulating pressure: You're at the side of the table, facing the client's spine, in a parallel foot stance. You're doing light pressure in the lamina groove so you need to hold back some of your body weight. Instead of letting your back take the brunt of the workload, you lean into the table with your thighs.

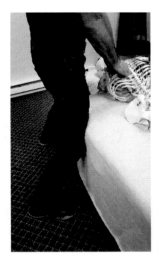

(2.2)

Moving between foot stances and how you lean into the table should be as fluid as changing massage strokes. If you're leaning with both legs against the table and it's suddenly not working, switch to another position, like one leg against the table.

There is no perfect stance to do an entire massage in, but there are better stances for particular situations. Moving into the best stance for your body to meet the demands of a particular massage situation is like a cool dance but without the jazz hands.

I just showed you leaning against the table with the fronts of your legs; how about leaning against the table with the side of your leg? That's something I never imagined that I'd be doing. But it's a key leg leaning technique for me now, especially when I'm doing one-handed massage. When you lean using the side of your leg into the table you won't be facing the client.

Okay, you know to lean a leg into the table to support your back. Now it's time to regulate your pressure by directing some or all of your body weight into the table and/or into the client.

Using the Massage Table to Regulate Pressure

Here are some basic guidelines for leaning into the table to regulate pressure.

For deep pressure direct all or most of your body weight into the client; medium pressure—half of your body weight into the client; and light pressure—25%.

Deep pressure is easy. Look out below, right? Well, not exactly, but you know what I mean—you're basically leaning all or most of your body weight into the client. But light and medium pressures are more nuanced. It may be 60% of your body weight into the table and 40% onto Maya. For Jorge it may be reversed, 40% of your body weight into the table and 60% of your body weight onto Jorge.

The art of leaning into your massage table starts with asking the "how's the pressure?" question to the client when you're leaning. Nailing the perfect pressure right off the bat doesn't take long to develop once you start getting your reps in.

You adjust your pressure by shifting your weight to the leg that's leaning into the table or to the body part that's doing the massage on the client. As you do this you may have a Zen moment where you realize that you're no longer using your upper-body to regulate pressure. Instead you're using your lower body.

To get to this Zen moment instantly I imagine what would happen if someone pulled the table out while I was leaning. Mark go boom. That is, if Mark is leaning with all his body weight he should go boom.

Even with light pressure?

Yep, my face should hit the floor even with light pressure because I should be leaning most of my body weight into the table. You might be wondering how falling on my face Zens me out. Well, falling on my face doesn't, but the image of letting myself lean and relax enough to fall does.

Close your eyes. Pick the body part that you are going to use to massage. It could be your forearm, elbow, fists, knuckles, fingers, or palms. Position that body part so that it's the landing gear for your touchdown on the client's body. Now see yourself gently falling into the client and/or table with all your body weight.

The only thing you need to do is direct the fall. For light pressure you're sinking into the table. For medium pressure you're sinking into the table and client. For deep pressure you're sinking into the client. No strain. Just sinking and directing.

That mindset takes some practice, and don't get hung up on the Zen part. You can deliver perfect pressure through leaning without Zen-ing out.

Pressure Governors

An easy way to make sure that you're consistently nailing light and medium pressure is to apply a governor, something that won't allow you to exceed the pressure you want to achieve.

For instance, if I'm in a narrow stance, feet close together, I have a lot of leaning distance between the client and me. If the table is low enough I can transfer all of my body weight into the client and/or table.

But a wide stance does what? It puts the body part that you are massaging with closer to the table and/or client, which means you have less leaning distance between the client and yourself than you would in a narrow stance. Therefore, you can't transfer all of your body weight into the client and/or table in a wide stance. The only way to do deep pressure in a wide stance is to muscle through the massage which is something that you triple promised me you weren't going to do. (See picture 2.2 in this chapter.)

So, a wide stance is a governor preventing the massage therapist from applying deep pressure in a "leaning to generate pressure" scenario.

Another governor is sitting.

When you sit and lean you're transferring the weight of your torso into the client and/or table. When you stand and lean you're transferring the weight of your entire body into the client and/or table. So, if you're sitting to generate pressure, you can only generate light to medium pressure when leaning.

To give you a visual that shows the governors in action, picture yourself sitting to massage a client's foot. Your client is prone and you're at the foot of the table, sitting on a stool. You lean into your client's arch with your thumbs.

Your client says, "That feels great, but could you go deeper?"

Well, from the seated position you have already leaned with the entire weight of your torso and maxed out how much pressure you can generate from leaning. So, you stand up and put a knee on the table and lean into your client's arch with your knuckle. Now you are using the weight of your torso and some of your lower body to generate pressure.

You're at medium to deep pressure and your client says, "That feels wonderful, but could you go a little deeper?"

Okay, but you've maxed out how much pressure you can generate in this one-knee-on-the-table position, so you stand. Standing allows you to transfer all your body weight into the client and/or table. You lean all your body weight into the client's arch. "Perfect," she says.

Regulating pressure through leaning does have a learning curve, but the good news is that you already know how to sit to massage, put a knee on the table to massage and stand to massage. Now, you just have to think about these positions as ways to regulate pressure. Personally, my favorite governor is my butt on a massage stool.

Now I have to admit that my relationship with my massage stool was not all chocolates and roses. In fact, for about 10 years I didn't have a massage stool in my massage room.

Yes, I'm cheap, but that wasn't the only reason I didn't have a stool in my massage room.

I thought that not sitting would make me stronger, tougher and a more durable massage therapist. Spoiler alert: It didn't. In fact, it made my pain issues worse. It was only during my year-long experiment that I discovered the massage stool not only helped me regulate pressure, but it also could help save my body.

How?

A massage stool allowed me to rest my (1) legs, (2) back, (3) shoulders, and (4) arms.

That's a lot of resting, huh?

Well, by now you can probably see that my massage hardening philosophy has taken a 180 degree turn over time. Now it's: Toughen your body in the gym, on a trail or in the water; preserve your body in the massage room.

Sitting on a stool is a way to give overworked muscles a rest break. Resting your legs is a no-brainer. You sit down on the stool and your legs say *aaaaah*. But what about resting your back?

Use a Massage Stool to Rest Your Back

It's easy. Pull up a massage stool and put your butt down. And if you really want to rest your back, use your arm-rests—your thighs. Here my forearms are on my thighs and my back is happy to be in a different position and to have the extra support of my forearms on my thighs.

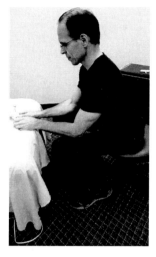
(2.3)

And to apply pressure effortlessly I just lean in from the waist with my forearms on my thighs. Couldn't be any easier. How about shoulders and arms? Same formula as back. Sit. Rest forearm(s) on your thighs. Lean.

That really takes the upper trap and levator scapulae out of the contraction zone.

What if your "armrests" are too low? Raise your stool or if your stool is at the top height, raise your thighs by pushing up to tiptoes while staying seated. I've also found it easy to sit and lean when working the IT band, peroneus longus/ brevis, and tibialis anterior.

Alright, time to experiment with leaning.

1. Get a friend to practice on who will give you honest feedback about pressure.

2. If you already lean to apply pressure, then you know what that feels like at your normal table height. So, pick a higher or lower setting to try. If you don't lean to apply pressure, start with your normal table height before you experiment with a lower or higher table.

3. Choose the body part that you use to massage the most with or one that you want to add to your toolkit.

4. Lean and direct your body weight onto the person on the table and/or into the massage table.

5. Do light and medium pressure by directing some of your body weight into the table.

6. Do deep pressure by directing most of your body weight into the person on the table.

7. Use the table for support.

8. Lean while sitting.

For additional help check out the free, instructional "how to lean" videos at www.painfreemassagetherapist.com. When you come back I'm going to show you how to lean and move using a technique I call "short stroke massage."

CHAPTER THREE

Short Stroke Massage

Let's take a step back to get perspective. You now put your own mask on first by asking "How do I get the job done without being in pain?" before and during each massage. That puts you in the mindset of taking care of your body when you massage.

You've also practiced using your body weight to generate pressure through leaning. Leaning takes the strain out of your neck, shoulders, arms and back because you no longer have to muscle your way through the massage.

As part of leaning, you've learned how to use the table to support your back and to regulate pressure. So you know how to lean effectively and efficiently, but you may have noticed that at this point you're basically doing acupressure or ischemic compression. If you want to be able to lean to deliver pressure throughout the massage you need to be able to move (glide) while leaning. That's what we're going to cover now.

Leaning has a built-in problem when you start to move, which is that if your body weight is directed into the table and/or client, how do you move your body and maintain a consistent massage stroke from point A to point B, while maintaining stacked joints (which shortens your "reach")?

For example, let's say you're facing the table by the side of the client and want to do a forearm deep pressure massage stroke from L5 to C7.

You lean on your forearm in the lumbar lamina groove and start to glide without moving your feet. At about T12 your shoulder and elbow are not in alignment. You're still leaning with all of your body weight and you feel a slight pressure in your shoulder. What do you do?

Option one: Keep your feet still and continue to overextend your shoulder. Option two: Stop the stroke, move and start the stroke again.

Option one—continue to overextend your shoulder—is the obvious no, but option two—stop the stroke, move and start it again— doesn't seem like a great alternative because the massage stroke is going to be choppy and not relaxing.

Fortunately, there's a way to use option two without making the massage stroke choppy. I call it "short stroke massage".

During the beginning of my experiment to massage pain-free, I noticed that my chronic shoulder condition kicked up when I stood at the head of the table and glided with both hands to the base of the sacrum. That move overextended my shoulder.

It was tough for me to come to terms with this observation, since the big, reach-glide stroke from the head of the massage table was a signature move for me. It went something like this: I observed that my shoulder clicked after I did the long, glide stroke. So, I was a good boy and stopped doing the stroke. And it worked, my shoulder felt better.

But then I thought, "Dude, you're not that old. You can handle that stroke." So I did it again—and my shoulder, once again, hurt. Like before, I stopped doing the move and my shoulder felt better.

That went on for a few more rounds until I realized that since that was a signature move, I couldn't just cut it out of my relaxation massage routine—I needed to replace it.

Standing at the side of the table with double fists seemed like a good glide option. And it was. My shoulder felt better. Notice I said "better", but not "pain-free". Even though I was leaning and my two fists together were acting as a brace for my shoulders, I was still over-extending at the end of the stroke.

Aha, this is where Mark came up with a solution for overextending his shoulder, you might think.

Nope.

I kept tweaking my shoulder because I was taught that an uninterrupted stroke (e.g., gliding from the upper back to the lower back without stopping) is super relaxing to the client. And my experience on the table reinforced my training that continuous strokes were incredibly relaxing.

It was only after about a month of shoulder tweaking that I was forced to put my shoulder ahead of a massage tradition. I knew that pain occurred when I was doing a long, back stroke from the side of the table with my fists.

When exactly did it hurt?

From the middle to the end of the stroke when I had to stretch and my shoulder and elbow joints *weren't* stacked.

Hmm…what if I broke the continuous stroke rule? So, when my shoulder would start to feel overextended, I would reposition my feet before I continued on.

Fortunately, I had seen the pause/small step move demonstrated in the video where Edward Mohr showcased Sandy Fritz's body mechanics principles, and I wasn't going into my massage experiment blind.[10]

So, I tried it once, just once, with a client, Ashira, and I waited for the lightning bolt. You know that lightning I'm talking about: I hate your massage and I think you suck and I'm never coming back. But there was no lightning bolt. In fact, Ashira went out of her way to tell me how much she loved the massage.

Okay, I thought, but that was only one sneaky stroke during a 60 minute massage. I was sure that the rest of my clients would object once I started using this new technique regularly.

Good-bye, massage. Hello, job I hate.

But as I tested it out, clients seemed to love it. This encouraged me. So I started to experiment with pausing many times during a stroke (sometimes 5 or 6 times). Again, I didn't lose a client—and my shoulders felt great.

Why did my shoulder feel great?

By moving my feet, I was ready to start up the stroke again with my work directly in front of me which meant I was in a position to efficiently and effectively lean into the client with my body weight and my joints aligned.

I tested the short stroke out on MTs and got the same positive reaction. Both the continuous and short stroke were relaxing. So, if it wasn't the continuous movement of a stroke that made the client relax, what was it?

I don't know for sure, but my guess is that it has to do with maintaining consistent pressure. If the pressure is the same during the glide phase as it is during the non-glide (pause) phase, then the person on the table is probably less likely to notice or care that a pause has happened.

Additionally, my Spidey senses tell me that perfect pressure overrides stroke type in this way: A client is more likely to put up with almost any stroke if the pressure is spot on for relaxation, but I don't think the fanciest stroke in the world would ever cancel out pressure that is NOT relaxing to the client.

A point to note: With short stroke massage you can create the feel of a long, continuous stroke by shortening the pause in between strokes. Conversely, you can lengthen the pause and really slow the pace of your massage down.

Short Stroke Recipe

Okay, let's try short stroke massage. First, let's segment a normal back stroke from base of neck to sacrum into 3 parts: upper (C7 – T4), middle (T5 – T12) and lower (L1 – L5). I actually segment the stroke even more, but segmenting the back into 3 parts is a good way to keep things simple in the beginning.

Next, pick a side of the table and choose the body part(s) (fingers, thumbs, knuckles, fists, elbows, forearms) you want to use for the short stroke.

Then pick a stance: (1) asymmetrical feet (lunge) or (2) parallel feet. In the asymmetrical stance, the back leg is locked.

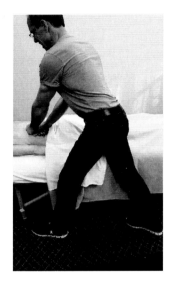

(3.1)

In the parallel stance both legs can be straight.

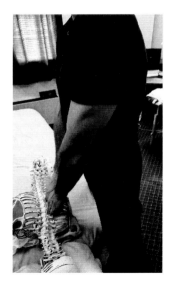

(3.2)

Next, start to glide, but pause when you feel yourself losing leaning leverage. *Don't* lift the body part you are massaging with off the client and *do* maintain the same pressure you were gliding with as you move your feet.

It's important to focus your attention on the body part you're massaging with (e.g. hand) because it's the connecting point to the client, and you don't want the client to sense a break in connection from you.

How you move your feet is up to you. I usually take a small step to get in position for the next short glide. Sometimes I twist my feet to move myself along.

How long you pause to get in position before you start the next short stroke is up to you also. Depending on the type of massage (focus or relaxation massage) my pause can be very short, like a second or two, or long, even minutes, if I've found something I want to focus on.

Start the next short stroke at the same relaxing stroke pace as you do with any long stroke. Resist the urge to speed up. Rinse and repeat up and down the back. By the way, you can do short stroke massage anywhere on the body.

Like anything new, short stroke massage will feel awkward at first, but once you experience the leverage advantage of moving your feet to get in position to lean efficiently and effectively, there's no turning back. And the pause that initially may seem disruptive to your flow can actually be part of a rhythm that slows you down and is a trigger for you to relax as you work.

Here's the Cliff's Notes to short stroke massage:

1. Pick a side and a stance.

2. Pick a body part to massage with and put it down on the client.

3. Lean and glide.

4. PAUSE when you start to lose leaning leverage.

5. *Don't* lift the body part you're using to massage and *do* maintain consistent pressure as you move your feet to reposition yourself.

6. Resume the next short stroke at the same relaxing stroke pace.

You can watch a free, short stroke video at www.pain-freemassagetherapist.com.

To recap, leaning to generate force is the foundation for massaging pain-free because when you use your body weight to generate pressure you're taking your upper-body out of the strain game.

The way you incorporate leaning into your massage may be different than the way I do it. That said, you'll have to experiment with leaning and figure out the best application for you.

But, Mark, what if leaning alone doesn't take care of all my pain issues or only helps by 50%, what then?

The answer is that there are other strategies and techniques to explore and that's what we're going to cover next. We'll do this by breaking down pain issues into three categories: hands and wrists, arms and shoulders, neck and back. Let's start with making achy hands not achy.

Part 2

TAKING PAIN-FREE MASSAGE TO THE NEXT LEVEL

CHAPTER FOUR

Pain-Free Hands and Wrists

I added a WARNING to this chapter because my editor-wife, Lisa, threatened to quit if I didn't. The WARNING is: Don't be surprised if you find this chapter slightly or even a lot overwhelming because it's packed with a ton of information that I think is important for you to have, and you can't really take it all in just by reading it. You actually have to physically do it.

If you're ready to practice some of the pain-free hands techniques in this chapter, by all means, dive in. But if you're not at that point yet, you may want to skim the chapter for general information until you have the time you need to experiment with the specific suggestions. Yes, this chapter requires effort, but at the end of the day, if you put the work in, I think you'll find this information to be helpful for saving your hands and prolonging your career. Now back to your hands.

If you blew through chapters one through three to get to this one, I get it. Hands and wrists are often the first sacrificial lambs to the cause of getting the job done. But that doesn't have to be the case any longer.

You're now paying attention to your pain and are ready to do something about it. In addition, you're open to challenging rules that are bad for your body and experimenting with new strategies and techniques. So, let's make those hands feel better.

Picture yourself leaning into the client with stacked joints. Your shoulder is over your elbow and your elbow over wrist—but what about your fingers?

If they were completely aligned with your shoulder, elbow and wrist they'd be straight out and you'd be jabbing your fingertips into the client. Not only would you have trouble selling jab-y massage, your finger joints would be compromised trying to bear the weight of your body.

So how do you spare your fingers from overuse and stress injuries when leaning?

Sure, forearms and elbows can be great substitutes for hands, but what about the times smaller points of contact are more desirable, like for neck and feet? And what about when working on very thin people or people who want light pressure? Or what if you wanted more sensitivity or precision? Or what if using a forearm feels awkward or triggers your pain condition, like it does for me? Or what if you just wanted more options to save your hands?

I have some solutions. The first one is to combine body parts.

Combine Body Parts

A thumb is one body part. Two thumbs together are combined body parts.

A knuckle is one body part. Two hands together with knuckles down are combined body parts.

You get the picture. Take a body part that you're going to massage with and add another body part to it. That can mean that the body parts are next to each other, on top of each other and/or interconnected.

Body parts next to each other act as a brace. A common, braced, body-parts combination is double-barred thumbs.

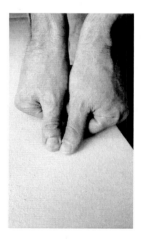

(4.1)

"On top of" means that instead of pressing with one body part, you're pressing with two. This spreads out the exertion effort and makes pressing easier. An example of "on top of" is thumb on thumb or a finger on a finger.

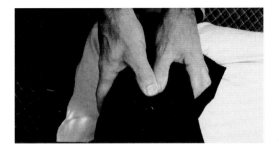

(4.2)

Interconnecting body parts adds stability and support to your fingers. A two-handed hold on a massage tool is an example of this.

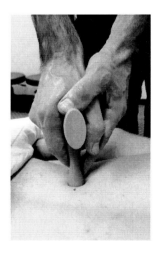

(4.3)

Massaging with combined body parts saves finger joints by providing support to finger joints. And if you're competent with body part combinations, you can switch out body parts during a massage so that you're not overworking any one body part.

Let's say you're a thumb-aholic and you're left-handed. After the third massage of the day your left thumb starts to ache and by the end of the day you're ready to quit massage.

But what if on massage # two you switched from using your left thumb exclusively to a knuckle-thumb combination or a double thumb combination? Now you are giving that left thumb some breaks throughout each massage. Less usage equals less wear and tear, and therefore, less pain.

I'm going to show you two of my favorite body part combinations. The first one is knuckle-thumb.

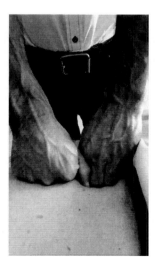

(4.4)

Knuckle-thumb is great for focus work because the knuckle and thumb together support each other and are small enough for detail work.

Do me a favor and take a look at the knuckle-thumb picture again. Do you see how my thumb is slightly flexed and braced by my middle knuckle of the other hand?

That's not an accident.

My fingers eventually figured out the best way to support each other. The flexion in the thumb prevents me from ramping up the pressure and overextending my thumb. Also, the middle knuckle on the other hand is acting like a support for that thumb.

By the way, I don't use my thumbs for focused pressure, aka, going after a trigger point. I use massage tools or knuckles for that. During a massage my happy thumbs are used to palpate and act as a sensing mechanism when I'm using a massage tool. So, it's rare if I exceed medium pressure with them and if I do, it's only for short burst. They primarily operate in the light pressure zone.

Here's my other favorite—knuckles-fist.

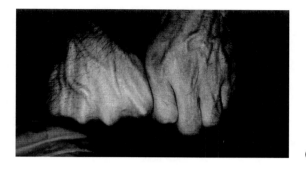

(4.5)

A knuckles-fist combination provides both focused and broad pressure. The middle knuckle of the knuckle hand is making the deepest contact with the client while the rest of the knuckles on the knuckle hand and the fist on the other hand are making broad contact.

This is a great body-parts combination for the erector spinae. My knuckles from one hand go in the lamina groove and the loose fist of the other hand "pushes" the knuckles from behind. In the picture above, the head of the person on the table would be to the right, in the dark area of the picture. The massage platform that is created between the two body parts is stable and relaxing. Sometimes you might even hear a spinal adjustment sound as you glide alongside the spine.

If you want even more of a generalized pressure feel, like you would get with a forearm, then you could use a double-fists combination instead of a knuckles-fist combination.

You can see how versatile combined body parts are in terms of providing focused or broad pressure. Here's one more that captures both focused and broad pressure in one move—the forearm-hand combination.

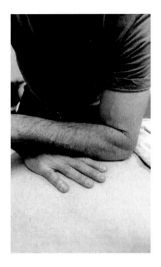

(4.6)

This forearm-hand combination is perfect for the MT who wants to use a forearm/elbow to replace thumbs. The hand is under the forearm and the thumb is being used as the sensing device.

What I love about this combination is that I'm not pressing with my thumb. My body weight is exerting the pressure. My forearm is the base that's receiving my body weight and I adjust how much pressure my thumb gets by where I place my thumb. Personally, I place my thumb so that the inside edge is receiving some of the pressure, just enough so that it can sink deep enough into the tissue below it and be a sensing device.

Go to www.painfreemassagetherapist.com for a free, "how to combine body parts" tutorial. Later I'm going to show you how to combine a massage tool and a hand. But now it's time to experiment.

Experimenting with Body-Parts Combinations

Start experimenting with any one of the combinations I just showed you. The goal is not for you to fall in love with the ones I like. The goal is to trigger your creative and adaptation responses so that you can figure out which combinations, variations and new creations work for your hands and body.

By the way, I don't think you'll find this to be a difficult process. Once you start to feel the power of bracing and interlocking body parts you'll find your hands looking for the most supportive positions. But I do need to tell you that this process can be addictive and extremely satisfying.

Satisfying?

Yep, that's the right word, but I'll need a pillow to explain what I mean.

Imagine, after 20 years, your favorite pillow finally gives up the ghost and you're forced to get a new one. You start looking and nothing is working. The pillow is either is too soft, too hard, too fluffy, not fluffy enough, too hot, too weird, too over-engineered, or not engineered enough.

What a pain. But you persevere and finally find a pillow that doesn't hurt your neck.

You can't wait to use your pillow and when you do you suddenly realize that your pillow journey is not over. You found a pillow that doesn't hurt your neck, but you still don't have a pillow that is perfect for your neck. In fact, the perfect pillow will probably require some squishing and squeezing and some bending and maybe even some punching until that perfect place in the perfect pillow is created for your head.

When you lay your head down in that perfect place in the perfect pillow what happens?

You sigh because the pillow is perfect for your neck.

That's the sigh you'll get the second you figure out the perfect body parts combinations for your hands.

Here's a sigh that I had recently. Kristin had taken my deep pressure class because doing deep pressure really hurt her back and hands. She wanted to practice on me because she was applying for a massage job.

Again, being the selfless person that I am, I agreed to be the one on the table who had to endure the parasympathetic relaxation response and the endorphin boost. At one point during the massage when I was prone I felt this incredibly deep, relaxing stroke on the side of my leg.

Wow, I said, *what's that?*

"I just made it up," Kristin said.

She put her hands next to the face cradle to show me her hand position. Her one fist was cupped in her other hand, and she was massaging, gliding, with the back of her cupped hand.

Immediately I stole her move and used it on my next client's IT band, but I added my own take on the move by sitting down.

Sitting took all the strain out of my back and acted as governor for my pressure.

Needless to say, I love my Mark's Massage Move Stolen From Kristin.

As you experiment with combining body parts you can also think about substituting body parts for body parts that you overuse.

Substitute Body Parts

Which body parts do you overuse?

I'm going to assume thumbs are high on your list. Thumbs are sturdy, sensitive and can get into tight spaces. But it doesn't take too many deep, focus-work massages to realize that thumbs weren't evolutionarily designed to be plunged into flesh.

Fortunately, there are thumb substitutes. A knuckle is one. And a massage tool is another.

Think about that rotation for a minute: thumb, knuckle, massage tool. How much better would your thumbs feel if you used them 2/3 less of the time when doing focus work? Add in body parts combinations, like barred thumbs, knuckle-thumb combo and a massage tool-thumb combo. Now we're off the charts with saving thumbs. And we're still not done. You can lessen wear and tear on your dominant thumb by using your non-dominant thumb, too.

Yes, you're still using thumbs, but you're spreading out the workload which can be huge in terms of giving your dominant thumb a break. But that requires you to become more ambidextrous.

Become Ambidextrous

Raise your hand if you're severely one-sided. I was. It felt unnatural and inefficient to use my non-dominant side. Why? Because it *WAS* unnatural and inefficient to use my non-dominant side. But with a little practice I got a little better and soon the idea of becoming competent with my non-dominant side didn't seem that farfetched.

This isn't exactly what I did, but I think it will get you to where you want to be. For the next 50 massages, every time you use a dominant-side body part for detailed work (e.g. left thumb), use a non-dominant-side body part (right thumb), too.

Make it easy when you first start by only placing a non-dominant-side body part down on the client for a few seconds. Gradually add more time. As you add time, explore with the non-dominant-side body part.

Why not?

We have the perfect work situation in which to experiment. We can eye the client for reactions. If you get a squirmy reaction, then stop, regroup and try in a different area later on in the massage, or try again with a different client. If you start racking up squirmy reactions, practice your non-dominant body part work on friends or at home with family.

Don't discount getting your reps in at home because they don't simulate a work setting. You are still building a connection in your brain that your non-dominant hand can do more than be non-dominant.

One of my favorite non-dominant things to do is to eat with my left hand. So far, only minor puncture wounds from an errant fork, but nothing that required a bandage or medical attention. If the fork scares you try brushing your teeth or combing your hair with your non-dominant hand.

Developing your non-dominant hand is not only helpful in massage, it's helpful in life in general, like when you have no other option but to turn a screwdriver with your non-dominant hand.

So far, we talked a lot about thumbs because they're ideal pokers. But the other fingers, 2, 3, 4 and 5, can get equally beat up during a deep tissue massage.

How do you protect all fingers?

Well, you can start by NOT squeezing every muscle that can be squeezed. Squeezing is tough on finger joints because it involves sustained muscle contraction of hand flexors. And it's particularly hard to resist squeezing certain muscles, like upper traps, right? They seem made for squeezing, but it will become easier once you have an alternative for squeezing. I have one for you.

Upper-Trapezius Non-Squeeze Release

In neuromuscular therapy (NMT) training I learned a technique for releasing the deeper tissue of the upper traps.

The client is prone. With one hand you grasp the top edge of the trapezius so that your four fingers are wrapped around the superior, anterior edge and your thumb is on the posterior side of the upper trap.

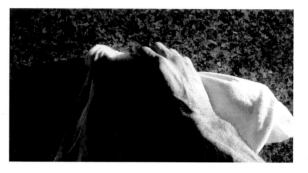

(4.7)

In this hand positioning you're going to grip the upper trap and then "unfurl" the trap edge by moving your fingers towards you and your thumb away from you, as if you're revving a motorcycle.

The goals of the NMT trap release are to deactivate hard-to-get-to trigger points and to change ischemic conditions in those areas. I don't subscribe strictly to NMT theory any longer, but I like the NMT trap release because it's pain relieving and relaxing to clients.

Unfortunately, I had two problems with the NMT deep tissue trap release. One, it beat up my hands. Two, my clients got used to it and loved it, and I felt stuck with it until I came up with a version that didn't hurt my hands.

Since squeezing and rolling with one hand was what caused hand pain when doing the NMT Upper-Trap Release, I decided to use two hands.

Look at the NMT squeeze picture (4.7). I replaced the thumb in the picture with a knuckle on my left hand, while my right hand still wrapped around the trap. Next, I pressed down with my knuckle into my fingers and I found that I could simulate the unfurling if I wanted to, without straining my fingers.

In addition, for clients with very thick upper-traps, I now add a massage tool which makes pressing even easier.

It's amazing how focused your pressure can get when pressing between two hands, and I think you'll have fun experimenting with calibrating your pressure using this technique. You can see a video of this technique at www.painfreemassagetherapist.com.

The "squeeze less" strategy and the use of "alternative squeezing techniques" are relatively easy to implement. Here's another hand-saving strategy that's a little more subtle: Relax your hands.

Relaxed Hands Strategy

The relaxed hand and I have a long history. When I was a massage student, a thousand years ago, I thought every MT had hand pain. My hands got to be such a problem that I went to my teacher, Telema, for help. She watched me work on a fellow student and within seconds she was tapping on my hands.

"Relax," she said.

They are, I reflexively responded.

She put her hand next to mine and did the same petrissage move I was doing. Now there was no denying that my white-knuckled hands were not relaxed. So, I copied Telema, and she walked away to check on another student.

When she came back she said, "Relax your hands."

We did a few more rounds of this before I could see when I was tightening my hands. Telema went off to check on other students and confident that I was relaxing my hand, I switched to using one hand to massage a neck.

Minutes later I felt someone tapping on my non-working hand Telema's voice say, "Relax your hand."

Damn it. She was right—I was tensing my non-working hand.

Relaxing the non-working hand was more challenging to recognize than the working hand, but eventually I got that, too. As time went on I realized that there was a hidden bonus to Telema's advice. The act of relaxing my hands became a trigger to relax my entire body. And when my body was relaxed I wasn't wasting energy.

There's a parallel between sports and massage here. If you're tense playing a sport, your performance will probably suffer. Can you think of a time when you played in a game, competed in an event or performed on stage where having a tense body helped? Probably not.

Okay, so you can't be Gumby and ooze all over the place. There needs to be a certain amount of tension in the right parts of your body. But excess tension wastes energy, is unnecessary and gets in the way of efficient execution.

Try this: Hold your arms out in front of you as if you were going to lean into someone on the massage table. Now make really tight fists. Do you feel the contraction of those hand, forearm, arm and shoulder muscles?

With the tightened fists, lean forward as if you're going to apply deep pressure to the glutes. Keep those fists tight! You should feel that your power (and strain) is coming from your arms and shoulders. That's a lot of muscle work going on.

Now, straighten back up. Keep the fists, but make them loose fists. Relax your forearms, arms and shoulders. Think of each arm, from loose fist to shoulder, as one connected unit. Now lean, but stay relaxed.

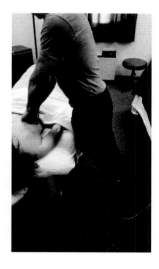

(4.8)

Where does your power feel like it's coming from?

It should feel like it's coming from your lean with no strain in your shoulders and arms. And you should feel like you're able to lean all your body weight easily.

In the picture it may not look like I'm relaxed, but trust me, I am. The relaxed lean is super-efficient and easy on your body, so easy you may find yourself closing your eyes, like X.

Admittedly, the next thing I'm about to say is going to sound strange. Relaxing my hands helps me with palpation. It's pretty simple. When I focus on relaxing my hands during a massage, my attention is on my hands. When my attention is on my hands, I become more aware of what I'm touching.

Additionally, relaxing my hands becomes an unconscious signal for me to relax my whole body.

There's one more hand-saving strategy that I need to talk about. It's the most powerful hand-saving strategy that I use, but there's a learning curve. It's massage tools.

CHAPTER FIVE

Massage Tools

No.

Yes.

No.

Yes.

Those are the answers to the most-asked questions I get about massage tools.

No, massage tools will not mess up the flow of your massage if you know what to do.

Yes, you can maintain sensitivity when using a massage tool if you know what to do.

No, you're not going to hurt anyone if you know what to do.

Yes, most people think massage tools feel good when you know what to do.

These are the exact questions I asked myself when I started using massage tools too, especially when I was doing a relaxation massage or relaxation/pain relief combination massage.

It wasn't always that way. When I was a neuromuscular therapist my expectations for making the massage feel good were low because my goal was to fix the client's problem. Period. The massage didn't have to be relaxing, flow-y or even quiet.

In fact, there was often a lot of talking.

On a pain scale of 1 to 10 what does it feel like when I press here?

"Six."

Ok. How about now?

And there were no smooth transitions from hands to massage tools. It was pick up the massage tool and plunk it down. But when using a massage tool became a way to save my hands in addition to being an extremely effective way to apply precise pressure, the game changed. I now needed to be sensitive with the massage tool when doing relaxation and pain-relief massage.

No plunking down the massage tool. My transitions from massage tools to hands and hands to massage tools needed to be smooth and relaxing or I would lose clients.

It took me many massages to figure out how to incorporate massage tools into every massage I did. My goal is to shorten the learning curve for you with this 3-step process.

How to Use a Massage Tool—3 Steps

Step #1: Have the table set at a height that allows you to lean efficiently and effectively.

We don't need to spend a lot of time on this step because we covered that in Chapter 2. But I do want to add this: If standing and leaning is not a strategy that is working for you, don't abandon sitting and leaning, especially with massage tools.

Working on a stool with a massage stool is particularly effective for feet and the tops of shoulders. You just need to figure out the best stool height for you to lean. Also, having a client take a side-lying posture will allow you to effortlessly use a massage tool on back muscles while you're sitting. Having the client closer to the edge of the table nearest you will prevent you from overreaching and stressing your arms and shoulders.

Step #2: Pin and lean the massage tool, then relax your hand.

You've learned how to lean to generate pressure in the previous chapters. Now you're leaning with a massage tool in your hand. Once you pin the massage tool between your hand and the client, you're then going to relax your hand.

Step#3: Add a guide finger for stability, to regulate pressure and to find areas you want to work. Steps one and two will save your hands. This last step will give you reassurance that you aren't going to jab clients with the massage tool.

Since we already covered leaning, step #1, in detail, let's start our deep dive into massage tools with step #2—pin and lean the massage tool, then relax your hand.

Pin, Lean and Relax

In NMT, I was taught to grip the massage tool so that my fingertips, specifically thumb, 2nd and 3rd fingers, were controlling the tip of the massage tool.

This fingertip grip gave me fine-tuned control of the T-bar when working a tight/tender spot, but it also encouraged me to grip the T-bar tightly, even when applying light pressure and over time that really hurt my fingers.

Hmm...what would happen if I just loosened my grip some?

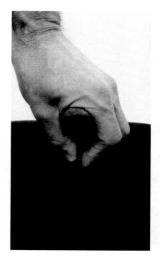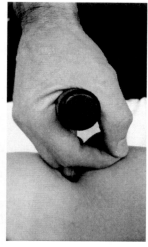

(5.1)

Nothing. The T-bar didn't slip out of my hand, and on a low table I could even open my hand because the tool was pinned between my hand and the person's body.

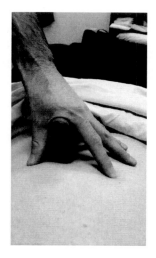

(5.2)

But there was still a glitch. When I tried to apply medium to deep pressure, my hand would start to tighten around the massage tool handle to steady the tool—and again I was gripping the massage tool like I had done in the past. Back to the massage room I went—specifically to experiment with the guide finger.

A guide finger is a digit, often a thumb, that is put next to a massage tool tip for sensing and palpating.

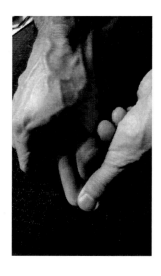

(5.3)

You find areas that you want to work and avoid with your guide finger. The importance of a guide finger can't be overstated. If you want to have and maintain sensitivity with a massage tool, you have to use a guide finger. After all, the guide finger is wired to your brain. The hunk of wood or slab of plastic—not so much.

Because a guide finger is placed right next to a massage tool it provides an additional benefit—it helps keep the massage tool upright. Taking note of that benefit, I doubled-down on making the guide finger a better massage tool stabilizer.

This wasn't hard to do. In fact, it was a lot of fun. I let my hands play until they found comfortable ways to stabilize a massage tool while maintaining contact with the tissue I was working on. When I did, interesting things happened.

I discovered a guide finger could be two fingers.

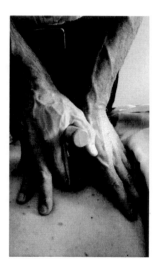

(5.4)

Or knuckles.

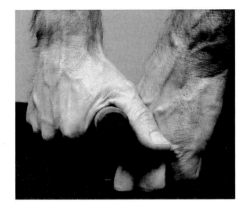

(5.5)

Or fists.

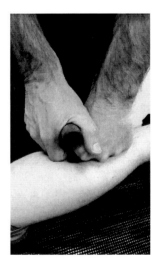

(5.6)

These guide finger positions provided a lot of support around the massage tool and when I leaned to apply more force, I didn't have to grip the massage tool harder. There are a lot more holds that I use, and you'll figure out your own as you experiment.

To keep it simple in the beginning, put a thumb from the non-holding hand next to the massage tool stem and let that be your guide finger. Get 100 reps in with a thumb guide finger. Once you do, you can experiment with other guide finger options. Be patient with this process. If you rush, you'll start making mistakes, like applying too much or too little pressure.

One last thing about a guide finger, if you want to press a trigger point or pain area with a specific amount of pressure, first press with your thumb (guide finger) to determine the appropriate pressure. Then apply the same pressure with the massage tool.

The "feel" that allows you to use a massage tool effortlessly and effectively takes some experimenting and lots of practice. So I'm not going to bog you down in details here. When you're ready to experiment with massage tools, go to www. painfreemassagetherapist.com for free, massage-tool tutorial videos.

Here's a quick recap of the massage tool basics: Pin the massage tool, lean, relax the hand holding the massage tool, and add a guide finger.

But before you can practice with a massage tool, you need to pick a massage tool. Here's how:

How to Pick a Massage Tool

Which is the best massage tool?

That's an easy answer: The massage tool that works best for you.

The harder question is: Which massage tool works best for you? To answer *that* question, you need to ask yourself three more questions:

1. Does the massage tool stress my hand when I use it for a few minutes?

In 2018, I wrote a massage tools article for Massage & Bodywork Magazine. I wanted to write exclusively about the T-bar because it was my go-to massage tool.

But the editor rejected that idea and asked me to do a comparative massage tools article. I went to the local massage supply store and played with the massage tools on display.

I eliminated 80% of the massage tools for the article simply by pressing them into the display table. If I had hand or wrist discomfort and couldn't figure out a way to hold the massage tool without producing discomfort—adios.

By the way, I didn't care if the packaging said "Voted Best Massage Tool for Feet" or "Designed by NASA Engineers!", if it hurt my hand, it hurt my hand. Period.

I should point out something here: If you become a massage tool addict like me, any hand-held massage tool is going to bother something (your palm, fingers or wrist) if you use it constantly or hold it too long. I'm going to explain how you counteract that in a second. For now just note that the massage tool that you *don't* want to buy causes immediate discomfort when you hold it AND scores low on question #2.

2. Can I hold the massage tool comfortably in multiple ways?

Basically, when you're using any massage tool you will need to mix up your holds. As I mentioned above, if you hold anything one way for a long period of time (even a pencil), you're going to over-stress certain joints and muscles. When you use different holds you spread the workload (and stress-load) out.

As you test out the massage tool that you're thinking about purchasing, try different holds. You don't need a body to work on. Just press that tool into a table or other surface. Does it hurt your hands? If so, can you find ways to hold it so that it doesn't hurt your hand?

I've found that a massage tool with a simple design, like a T-bar with a handle and one contact end, is easier to hold than a complex massage tool with multiple contact ends. Why? Because multiple contact ends means you have less places to actually hold the massage tool.

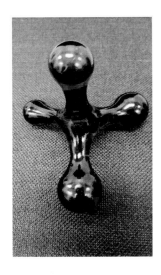

(5.7)

Here's the last question you need to ask yourself when buying a massage tool.

3. Is the massage tool only good for one pressure or can I use it for light, medium, and deep pressure?

A lot of massage tools are fine for light pressure, but for medium or deep, not so much. You may have noticed in the pictures that all the massage tools that I'm demonstrating have a handle. There's a simple reason for that. Massage tools with handles are ideal for leaning because they provide enough of a purchase to lean into.

I have 30 or so massage tools. I use 4 on a consistent basis, and 3 more on an occasional basis. The rest just take up storage space. If you buy a massage tool and it's not a winner, don't give up, you're now better informed to find the one that will be your homerun. (To see my favorite massage tools, go to www.painfreemassage.com).

If you can't decide which massage tool to go with, I'd go with the basic wooden T-bar because of it's versatility.

So, let's say you have your massage tool and you know what you're supposed to do with it. Now you need to practice.

Practicing with Your Massage Tool

When do you do that?

NOT on paying clients if you're brand new to massage tools.

After removing barriers to using massage tools, it may look like I'm erecting one now, but I'm not. What I'm trying to do is to set you up for success. You're not going to be successful if you take a massage tool into the massage room and expect to be successful at using it right off the bat, when the only feedback you'll get from the client is if they flinch or randomly say, "That feels good."

Plus, a client is paying for a massage *session*, not a massage *experiment* in which they are the subject of the experiment. Grab a massage therapist friend or someone you trust to give you instant and reliable feedback. Don't just settle for one opinion. Get as much reliable feedback as you can. I have the benefit of getting a lot of feedback from a lot of massage therapists when I teach my massage tools classes. That information has helped me become proficient and confident with massage tools.

Also, (shameless plug coming), buy a copy of this book for a massage therapist friend so that you can do exchanges. Then you get to be on the table, experiencing massage tool work firsthand. It's important to know what it feels like.

But seriously, you'll never feel comfortable using a massage tool if you don't get the feedback and put in the work to develop the "feel" necessary to hone your sensitivity. Practice done on appropriate volun-teers – and plenty of it – is key.

At some point as you practice with a massage tool, you'll arrive at the "Now what?" moment. The "Now What?" moment occurs when you feel okay using a massage tool on friends, but you're still hesitant to use a massage tool on a paying customer.

The "Now what?" moment can end your massage tool jour-ney without you realizing it. It's subtle. You have the mas-sage tool in the room with you, but you never pick it up and use it. Why? You still don't have confidence that you can use a massage tool in a way that doesn't make the massage feel awkward or ruin the massage for the client.

You take the awkwardness out of using a massage tool by getting good with transitions.

Massage Tool Transitions

I remember taking a particular NMT course and my partner for the day was a chiropractor. As you might expect, he knew anatomy inside and out and during that seminar he showed me some tricks of his trade for palpating and working near the spine.

I didn't feel I had much to offer him until I was the one on the table and he was the one practicing the NMT technique. He took the oil bottle, held it 6 inches above my back and squeezed. Oil oozed all over my back and then I felt his hands slap it around to keep it from dripping around to my front. What if you did that during a massage—how many clients would you have in your phone contact list?

Let's see…there'd be your mom, a friend who you massage for free and is too cheap to pay for a massage…oh, and the website designer you were supposed to barter with, but for some strange reason never had time to work on your website after you gave her the first barter massage.

How you introduce the massage tool to the client can NOT be the transitional equivalent of squirting oil on their backs from 6 inches away. In fact, the introduction should be seamless.

A lot of the time clients don't even know that I'm actually using a massage tool on them.

What's the secret to my sneakiness?

I keep one hand on the client as I pick up the massage tool. So the massage tool needs to be close enough for me to reach.

That contact hand is not a floater hand. I'm making firm con-tact with my client. There is intention, directionality, if you will, in my touch.

In other words, my brain is focusing on the contact hand as I transition to the tool. My client experiences that contact hand as me doing massage, and massage continuity is not broken.

The reverse is also true. If I'm transitioning from using a massage tool and want to put the massage tool down, I keep my guide finger/hand/fist on the client as I'm putting the massage tool down on the table.

That's it.

Once you get the hang of keeping a hand on the client when transitioning, you can then get super-efficient at getting the tool in and out of your hand smoothly.

In essence, my transitions have become part of my mas-sage pace which is slow and deliberate. Your pace may be different than mine. My point is that transitions should eventually feel as much a part of your massage as any technique you do in a massage. You can get to that stage simply by keeping one actively working hand on the client as you pick up or put down a massage tool. At that point, you're ready to use your massage tool on a paying client.

Now you've got all the information and free resources (www.painfreemassage.com) you need to experiment with massage tools.

Remember that using massage tools has a bigger learning curve than the other strategies, but you can shorten the curve by following the tips I gave you.

In the next chapter we're going to revisit leaning and how it can help with shoulder and arm pain.

CHAPTER SIX

Pain-Free Shoulders and Arms

I hate going to the doctor. Do you know what I do instead of going to the doctor? I ask Lisa to diagnose me.

Hey, Lisa, this brown mark on my head, it's not cancer, right?

"Go to the doctor," she says.

I often don't, and simply hope that whatever is bothering me goes away. A heads up for the younger MTs, this is not a good strategy for keeping yourself healthy in life or in the massage room.

The point is, if you have a shoulder or arm injury—or any injury for that matter—don't do what I do. Go see a doctor and get help. After that if you need to figure out a workaround for your shoulder or arm in the massage room, read on.

Review First

Let's first review what I've talked about already regarding shoulder and arm pain. In a 2010 study, Edward Mohr demonstrated that leaning to generate force was more effective than pressing to generate force. He also showed that stacking joints was easier on joints than non-stacked joints. Taking that together, it has been my experience that if I lean and stack my joints when massaging, my shoulder, elbow and wrist joints get happy.

I stopped triggering acute shoulder pain when I eliminated strokes that tweaked my shoulders. One stroke that bothered my shoulders was when I stood at the head of the massage table and glided all the way down to the client's sacrum. I also doubled-downed on short stroke massage. When I did, my shoulders could remain stacked as I leaned and glided.

A key change in my techniques to help with my persistent shoulder pain was switching from leaning on one forearm to leaning on two fists. Why? It was easier on a shoulder joint when both shoulders shared the workload to stabilize my body weight (leaning on fists) rather than just one (leaning on a forearm) having to do all the work.

Another change was to replace my elbow with a broad-tipped massage tool when doing trigger point work. This change helped to resolve the elbow pain (cubital tunnel syndrome) that I was experiencing at the time because I was no longer irritating my ulnar nerve when I pressed.

A broad-tipped massage tool not only helped resolve my elbow pain, it was easy on my shoulders. I did say shoulders, as in plural, and it's not a mistake. When I'm using a broad-tipped massage tool I have two hands on the tool. Two hands on the massage tool spreads out the workload between both shoulders and allows me to keep my shoulders in alignment as I lean to generate force.

Lastly in the review, I want to mention that I squeezed less and pressed more which meant less work for my shoulders and arms, especially if I was supporting my arms when leaning, like when I sat and leaned with my forearms on my thighs.

So far what I haven't talked about regarding eliminating shoulder and arm pain in the massage room is awareness. Being aware of pain is easy when your shoulder or arm hurts. The trick is to be aware of situations that could trigger your shoulder or arm pain in order to avoid them or mitigate their affect.

For instance, I noticed that a lot of my shoulder pain happened towards the end of the massage and towards the end of the work day. At those times I was more likely to overextend my shoulder or do a move that tweaked my shoulder because I was tired and getting lazy. A perfect example of that would be reaching instead of moving my feet to get in position to do the next massage stroke.

Knowing my vulnerabilities late in the day, I've taken these precautions: I talk to myself when I see that I'm getting tired. *Come on, Mark. You're reaching. Move your feet.* That's an automatic response in me now and is 90% effective, but not when I'm running on fumes. To avoid running on fumes, I take a preemptive approach and have snacks to eat in between clients so that I don't dip into the low brain glucose territory and start making bad decisions.

Now, let's look at two examples that show shoulder-and-arm-saving strategies/techniques in action.

Eliminating Forearm Pain Example

Sofia has terrible forearm pain and she's always looking to do exchanges with massage therapists. One day she decides to tackle her forearm pain head on. So she asks herself, "How do I get the job done without being in pain?"

First, she realizes that she is constantly squeezing, so she experiments with pressing substitutes. At the end of the day, she still likes to squeeze better than she likes to press, but is able to replace 50% of her squeezing with pressing.

Next she notices that her forearms hurt when she's massaging feet, but most of the time she doesn't notice them because her wrist and hands ache the most and get all of her attention.

She tries some body parts combinations on feet, but she doesn't feel much relief with her forearms. Then she tries a massage tool and almost immediately her hands feel better, but her wrists and forearms don't.

She tries different massage tools but they only marginally make her wrists and forearms feel better. She thinks it has something to do with the angle she's using the massage tool, so she experiments with her body position.

Instead of sitting and massaging feet, she puts a knee on the table so she can lean with her torso to generate pressure. Two things happen when she does that: (1) She can use more of her body weight to generate pressure, which means her forearm muscles now do less work. (2) In the knee-on-the-table position she can keep her wrist straight and she feels less strain in her wrist.

As Sofia gets better with leaning to generate pressure, she revisits the press move that replaced her squeeze move 50% of the time. She tries the press move with a massage tool while sitting with her arm supported. It's super easy on her forearms and now she's able to replace 90% of her squeeze moves with press moves.

Are you starting to get a feel for how eliminating pain while massaging is a process? One strategy or technique may work, while others may not. You just need to keep experimenting to figure out your pain-free formula.

Okay, Sofia is on her way to eliminating forearm pain. Let's address arm pain.

Eliminating Arm Pain Example

Joo has been doing massage for a while and has been married to his way of massaging. But now his arms ache. He knows there's a little biceps tendinitis going on, but he's okay with that—it's just the constant aching in his arms that's driving him nuts.

He starts to deconstruct his massage pain by looking for moves that make his arms stiffen and/or ache. It doesn't take him long to find one: The client is supine and Joo is reaching under the client's back with palms up, fingers digging into her rhomboids.

(Author interjection: Stop doing that!)

It's one of his signature moves and Joo doesn't want to give it up. He does it a lot. So he makes a deal with himself to reduce the time he does this signature move by 50%. It doesn't work because he can't restrain himself. It's all or nothing. But now he's aware that this move kills him and he has to stop doing it, so it has to be "nothing". But Joo has no idea what he's going to do to replace that move.

After having some time to get his head around the situation, he realizes that it's the body weight of the client that's putting all the stress on his hands and arms. What if he did the move with the client prone? Well, it would be hard on his fingers trying to generate that kind of pressure.

Joo then realizes that if he had the client prone or in a side-lying posture, he could really put some focused pressure into the rhomboids with a massage tool. It wouldn't provide the same sensation as the supine move, but it would allow him to target the rhomboids without putting himself in pain.

Clients like the super-focused work on their rhomboids and Joo's arms feel a little better at the end of the day. Joo continues to purge techniques that overuse his arms and replace them with ones that don't.

These examples are based in the reality of my experience. Your experiment will be different than mine. The common thread will be replacing techniques that cause you shoulder and/or arm pain and trying out some of the strategies and techniques that I suggested. You may end up with the same pain-free formula that I use, or yours may be a little different—or a lot different. It's all good. Getting out of pain is what matters, and that means being willing to find, acknowledge and change what's causing the pain to begin with.

In the next chapter I take the neck and back pain strategies/techniques I've talked about and plug them into real-life massage scenarios. I want you to see the thinking process involved in eliminating pain so that you can proactively engage in it yourself. I also explain two important concepts that could play into prolonged back and neck pain—perpetuating factors and staying in one body position for too long—and I show you how I deal with them so that I continue to massage pain-free.

CHAPTER SEVEN

Pain-Free Neck and Back

I dreaded when a new client and I would sit down to talk. The way our furniture was positioned in the office forced me to turn my head to the left to face the client, which made my left hand tingle. If I turned my head to a neutral position, it would stop. The tingling happened in the massage room too, where keeping a neutral neck was hard to do because of the many work positions I was in. I decided to pay attention to the times when my neck was most likely NOT to be in a neutral position, like when doing detail work where I really wanted to see what I was working on.

At first when I caught myself, I'd simply turn my neck so that it wasn't rotated and then I'd straighten my neck—but without straightening my back. However, this strained my posterior neck muscles because to straighten up from the neck only, I had to cock my head back. To fix this, I simply straightened my back *before* I straightened my neck. My back and neck loved having breaks from being in one position too long and craved more breaks.

I realize that finding opportunities in the massage room to stand upright ("get vertical") is not a ground-breaking discovery or earth-shattering news. But for me, "thinking about me in the massage room" was a big deal. And getting vertical was something that not only helped me eliminate neck and back pain, it just felt really good to do for both my mind and body.

By the way, I wasn't stealing time away from the client because I didn't stop massaging when I straightened my torso. I wasn't straightening up at the client's expense. In fact, I think that the recharge I get from taking a second or two to straighten my torso translates into a better massage for the client. After all, happy massage therapist = happy client, right?

How I "Get Vertical"

How I get vertical is simple. I just pay attention to my butt. When my torso is not over my butt, I'm not vertical.

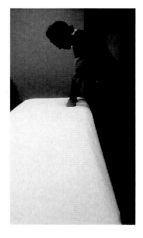

(7.1)

In this picture 7.1 you can see that I've slipped into a significant head-forward posture. I want to get vertical without stressing the back of my neck. So I'm going to bend my knees and let my thigh lean against the table. With my body weight being partially supported by the table it's easy for me to straighten my back and then my neck.

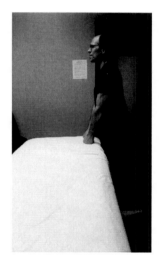

(7.2)

This works because, one, bending my knees keeps me low enough to my work so that I don't have to round my back and, two, my inner leg against the table helps support my body weight. In fact, any leg lean into the table gives you the opportunity to straighten up and break out of a bad posture.

How long do I straighten up for?

It depends. My vertical breaks are usually 2 to 3 seconds, but they could be for minutes if it makes sense—for example, if I'm doing focus work in a particular area while I'm vertical.

Often I get vertical when I transition from a two-handed massage stroke to a one-handed massage stroke. Here I'm doing a two-handed, short-stroke glide and my upper back is starting to fatigue because I've been in slight thoracic flexion for a while.

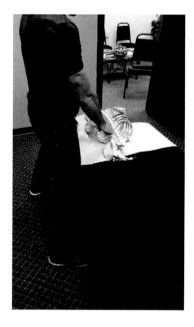

(7.3)

To get vertical I simply turn both feet to my right and lift my chest up and out—boy, does that feel good between my shoulder blades!—while switching to one-handed massage.

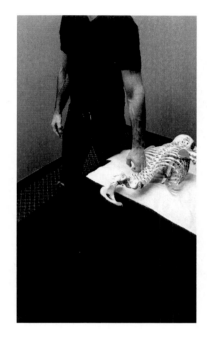

(7.4)

My feet are parallel to the side of the table, and I regulate my pressure through my stance. With a wider stance I have less leaning leverage. A narrow stance gives me more leaning leverage. If I want to give my working arm a break, I can turn the opposite way and use my other hand on the same spot or another spot.

Feet are also a time to get vertical. A wide stance allows me to get my butt under my torso.

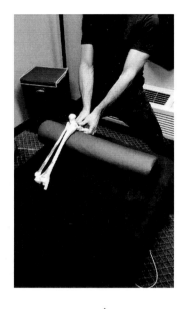

(7.5)

When you experiment with stances and one-handed massage, you'll find your own opportunities to get vertical. Here's a more complex move that still has good, vertical, massage body-mechanics.

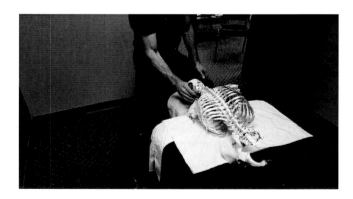

(7.6)

I'm using a T-bar on the upper trap/levator scapulae (or where the upper trap and levator scapulae would be if my skeleton was a person). To rest my shoulder and neck, I have my arm against the front of my torso, and I'm applying pressure by simply pushing with my legs, not my shoulder. (*Whisper voice: Lisa says I don't look so relaxed in the picture, but I am.*)

You can also take "getting vertical" a step further and stretch. To be clear, I'm not talking about breaking out the yoga mat and getting into cobra. I'm talking about taking advantage of an opportunity during a massage where extending your spine is possible without disrupting the massage.

After all, we spend so many of our working hours in spinal flexion. Counteracting all that flexion with a moment or two of deliberate extension is a healthy thing to do. Do it. As long as you don't interrupt or change your client's experience of the massage, you aren't short changing them in any way. The client is still the highest—but not the only—priority in the massage room. It's okay to take care of both of you. That said, while there is nothing wrong with a quick stretch, it could look odd to your client, so I'd only do it while they're prone.

The most basic stretch is to raise one arm in the air. Try lifting your torso as you raise your arm. Your back will love that.

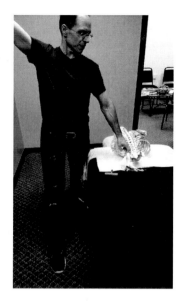 (7.7)

For more on getting vertical and stretching in the massage room, check out the free videos at www.painfreemassagetherapist.com.

We just looked at how getting vertical in the massage room could help with neck and back pain. Now, I want to specifically focus on back pain by going through an example with an MT.

Eliminating Back Pain Example

Shanice's back pain comes and goes, but now that she's increased the number of massages she does a week it's become persistent. The pain is low—lumbar and SI—and ranges from a dull ache to a sharp pain that is starting to wake her up at night.

She doesn't want to cut back on her massage because she's applying for a house loan in a year and wants bigger numbers on her tax return. Shanice starts to watch when her back pain occurs and intensifies in the massage room.

Her observation is that her back pain seems to flare up when she's doing deep pressure and intensifies as the day goes on. She starts her experiment with deep pressure using her fists on her friend's back and lowers her table two notches. Instantly she feels that it's easier to do deep pressure, so she lowers the table even more.

She uses the table for support, but the table height she's at now is not working for her body, so she puts her table back to her first experimental height, two notches from her normal height and instead of fists she tries forearms.

This is easy on her body. One, the table is supporting her body better than it did when she was using her fists and, two, she has great leaning leverage and it's easy for her to do deep pressure. All's good, but when she gets to the glutes, the way she has to position her body to use her forearm bothers her back again.

At this point she tries a T-bar with a fist as a brace and guide. That doesn't bother her back when she does glute work straight on; however, when she gets to gluteus minimus she has to adjust her stance and that bothers her back.

She figures she just needs to be in a position that doesn't strain her body for the gluteus minimus work and she will have the glute massage down pat. So, she sits down and leans into the gluteus minimus with a large, round-tipped massage tool. That works.

After she's done the buttock she continues to sit on her stool because sitting feels like it's giving her back a rest. She works the IT band by leaning and using a body parts combination technique, fist in palm.

She stands up to do the hammies and leans in with fists. She chose fists because leaning with her forearm would mean that she would have to go lower than she did when leaning with her forearm to massage her client's back—and that might be too low and irritate her back.

Leaning with her fists in the hammies is perfect for her back. She doesn't need to lean real hard to generate enough pressure and her arms are acting as supports to the point where she can straighten up her back. Her back is feeling better and she leans her body weight into the table with her legs so that she can get her torso vertical for a few seconds.

At her friend's feet she's back on the stool. She barely has to lean at all to generate the appropriate pressure for the points she wants to hit in her friend's arch using a round-tip T-bar.

Shanice continues the massage by adjusting what she does as she goes. Here's what she learned: Her back pain goes away or is less when she: (1) leans with a forearm on higher ground, like backs, (2) uses fists in valleys, like hamstrings, (3) sits on a stool and leans and (4) uses massage tools strategically to reduce the effort involved to produce focused pressure.

She takes this formula into the next massage and continues to tweak it. As her back improves she continues to adjust her formula to emphasize prevention rather than intervention.

For instance, she may start to add vertical moments during the massage to give herself breaks from times she reverts to bent posture, or she may choose to sit more on long days to avoid too much time on her feet, which could trigger her back pain.

Perpetuating Factors

Before I talk about the next example, I want to introduce a concept that has been very important to getting me out of pain in the massage room—perpetuating factors.

The bible for NMT is Travell and Simons' *Myofascial Pain and Dysfunction: The Trigger Point Manual*, Volumes 1 and 2. Though not cheap, I think the detailed muscle drawings alone make these manuals worth the investment. A new client doesn't get out my door without seeing a picture of the number one muscle that is causing her grief. Travell and Simons also cover perpetuating factors extensively in these manuals. For the purposes of keeping massage therapists out of pain, I've taken their definition of a perpetuating factor and modified it.[11]

I define a perpetuating factor as anything one does or has that causes, aggravates or prolongs pain. The "does" could be anything from bad work posture to bad decision making. The "has" could be an imbalance or a condition.

In NMT we looked for perpetuating factors that were structural, like a short leg or a hemipelvis. These perpetuating factors could cause persistent pain syndromes. For example, if you have a short leg and stand, your body will tilt and then compensate (make adjustments to rebalance). Sometimes those adjustments could create pain syndromes.

That made a lot of sense to me, and I was all in. I armed myself with scales, goniometers, markers and charts, and I went to town figuring out the structural perpetuating factors that were trashing my clients' bodies. But then one day I injured my back.

No problem, I thought, I'll just figure out my structural perpetuating factors and fix myself.

I carried a tape recorder so that I could record all my pain observations, hoping to find clues that would lead to my improvement, but nothing stood out.

I stood on two scales every morning and night and recorded my weight distribution numbers, but found no consistent imbalance between my sides.

I called my friend Heather who is a chiropractor and we set up appointments. Heather took X-rays of my spine and found no structural imbalance. She adjusted me for weeks and I didn't improve.

I also went to a McKenzie physical therapist and followed a back rehab script. She said that I didn't have a gait imbalance or a leg length differential and that my arches were fine.

I hired the massage therapist who was working for us at the time to give me deep pressure massage. He didn't find any area in my back that seemed to be the locus of my pain.

I was baffled and I wasn't getting better. In fact, I was getting worse. A lot.

Finally, in desperation, I stopped everything, both searching for structural perpetuating factors and all treatments. And within a month I was better.

Over the next year, I began to understand what had happened. Initially, I had tweaked my back working out. Then I made things worse by trying to fix it with aggressive treatments and continuing to massage without making adjustments in the massage room to reduce my current back pain. *I was the perpetuating factor.*

As I flipped to the 10X lens of the microscope I saw more times during that back pain episode when I'd failed to address a perpetuating factor, and I began to realize that addressing lifestyle/mindset (non-structural) perpetuating factors could not only help me *get* out of pain, they could also *keep* me out of pain.

Before I talk about how addressing perpetuating factors can get/keep you out of pain, I need to fess up. I just told you that the aggressive rehab and my stubborness were the perpetuating factors that kept my back from feeling better, but I left out the worst one. Why? It's embarrassing.

I continued to work out like a fiend even though my back hurt. How? I did substitute exercises, but I didn't turn down the intensity. For example, if heavy leg press hurt my back a particular day, I would substitute in something like sprinting on a treadmill at the highest incline. Guess what? That hurt my back, too.

It was only after I stopped all aggressive rehab AND intense workouts for a month that my back got the break it needed and started to mend. As I mended and got a little wiser (just a little) I started to wonder how I could avoid back pain in the future, and I realized that I might be able to avoid back pain if I set my radar to detecting lifestyle/mindset perpetuating factors too.

When I did, I started to uncover patterns of thinking and being that were putting me in the injury zone. One pattern was what I call whack-a-mole mindset. Here's an example of the whack-a-mole mindset. I used to work on my obliques by doing twisting leg raises from side-to-side. That meant I was on my back with my legs straight up in the air and perpendicular to my torso. I would swing my legs side-to-side, all the way to the floor, without touching the sides of my feet to the floor. Sometimes after long work days outside—I had a gardening business and massage business at the time—I would hear a pop and I could barely get up. You'd think that I'd stop doing this exercise at least when I'd had really physical days at work, right? But no, I wanted to do what I wanted to do.

It took many pops before I was willing to let that exercise go and replace it with an obliques exercise that didn't hurt my back, like side crunches. But I still only get partial credit.

Great, I'd think, *side crunches don't aggravate my back, let's add some weights to these puppies.* Then my back would go pop again. Do you see how this whack-a-mole game plays out?

I would substitute an exercise that didn't hurt my back, but then I'd increase the intensity of the exercise until it did hurt my back, which would send me off to find a new exercise. This mindset was a hard one to rewire. In fact, there was no rewiring. Instead, after many years of being stuck, I created a workaround to save me from myself.

I accepted that left to my own devices in the weight room I will eventually injure myself because I would keep heaping on more exercises. The workaround was to not give myself enough time to hurt myself in the weight room. Instead of giving myself an hour plus, I cut back my workouts to 30 minutes max. That worked at first, but ultimately it required that I be good and abide by the rule, and eventually workout brain was like, *Yeah, we're not doing that.* So I set up guardrails.

Guardrail number one was to squeeze a workout in between things in my schedule that had hard start and finish times so that I only had 30 minutes to work out.

Guardrail two: I stopped counting. If I never knew exactly how many reps I was doing it would be impossible for me to set up a comparison between workouts which was often a source of pushing myself to a breaking point—You did 9 reps last workout, you have to get 10 today (subtext: even if you have to cheat and break form).

The last guardrail was to stop taking copious notes about my workouts. Notes reinforced counting and increasing weight.

Today I take the tack that if I'm not having fun working out, there's something wrong. And if I'm dreading a workout because there's a burgeoning injury or pain issue, then it's time to take a break.

I talked about my mindset in the gym to give you an idea of how deeply a perpetuating factor may be ingrained. Here's one more example to get your brain thinking about lifestyle/ mindset perpetuating factors that may be affecting *your* neck and/or back in the massage room.

Terry has a bit of a martyr syndrome going on. When he's in the car with his wife, Layla, on a long trip, he won't let Layla have a turn behind the wheel even though Layla volunteers many times.

Halfway home on a 7 hour drive, Terry feels his sciatica starting to act up, but instead of stopping for a break or let- ting Layla take a turn driving, he pushes on.

Layla notices Terry getting squirmy and again offers to drive, but Terry shakes her off. When they're about 30 minutes from home, Terry can barely take the pain, and punches the accelerator when the stoplight turns green. Layla's neck is not happy with that jackrabbit start and they finish the drive in silence.

The next day in the massage room Terry's butt is on fire and sitting on the stool makes his sciatica even worse. So for the rest of the week he stands when doing massage, but standing triggers his all too familiar plantar fasciitis. With a constant electrical feeling down his leg, numbness in his foot and a stabbing pain in his heel, running is out of the question for the next week or so.

Terry is frustrated and racks his brain to figure out what went wrong. Perpetuating factors are sometimes hidden behind mental walls, like Terry playing the martyr behind the wheel. Other people can sometimes help us see them. Consider listening to people who you trust and have good insights about you. They could be pointing you in a direction that uncovers a perpetuating factor that has tripped you up for years.

There's one more thing that I want to say about perpetuating factors. Besides getting you out of pain and keeping you out of pain, understanding perpetuating factors may save you time and money.

Lorenzo was a client of mine who would come to see me when his lower back acted up, maybe 2 – 3 times a year. One time he came in with extreme pain in an area by his right, upper scapula and the front of his shoulder. It was a completely new pain.

He said that there was no event that caused it and nothing had changed in his activities at home, work or play.

His guess was the he reinjured the rotator cuff that he'd had surgically repaired a couple of years ago. But that didn't add up because his range of motion was fine in that shoulder and there was no strength loss. Maybe there was a perpetuating factor.

In the massage room, Lorenzo yelped when I pressed the pain area, but from a palpation standpoint the pain area felt the same as the side that didn't bother him. I went back to asking questions and I got the same response—nothing has changed.

Lorenzo thought some more and after a few minutes said, "Well, I did change my desk."

Lorenzo's new desk was a standing desk. The standing desk fit on top of his current desk. He adjusted it up when he stood to work. He lowered it when he sat down.

When he stood to work, his arms were completely unsupported and his shoulder and upper back had to do more work. It could be that under the added muscular strain, his right shoulder/scapula area (compromised from being injured before) rebelled. In addition, the pain began at the same time he changed to the standing desk.

Also worth mentioning, is that Lorenzo jumped into standing almost 100% of the time, instead of mixing it up, like standing 50% of the time and sitting 50% of the time. I suggested cutting back on the standing time, but Lorenzo decided to eliminate the standing desk altogether and the pain went away.

What if Lorenzo hadn't addressed the standing desk as a perpetuating factor for his upper-back pain? His medical trajectory may have been a doctor's visit, muscle relaxants, anti-inflammatory pills or an X-ray and if need be, an MRI and injections. In other words, a lot of time and expense without a potential perpetuating factor being addressed.

In the examples, we've talked about perpetuating factors for backs, but I'm sure it's obvious to you that the search for perpetuating factors can and should be applied to any pain condition anywhere on your body.

I find if I keep these 3 questions in mind when looking for a lifestyle/mindset perpetuating factor, I have an excellent chance of figuring things out:

1. Has anything changed in work, home or recreational life?

2. If so, when did the change occur?

3. If just before or soon after the pain occurred, could this change be connected to the pain?

And remember, as you turn your lens inward, it's possible that you're filtering out something that's important, but you think isn't, like Lorenzo did with his standing desk (by assuming that a standing desk was going to be good for him).

As the physicist Richard Feynman once said, "The first principle is that you must not fool yourself, and you are the easiest person to fool."[12]

I can attest to that.

One final thought about perpetuating factors. Look at this list:

► Refusing to put on your own mask first (prioritize your pain).

► Subordinating your physical comfort to "rules" and traditions.

► Clinging to techniques that hurt you because new ones feel awkward and different.

► Clinging to techniques that hurt you because everyone else does them.

► Never giving new techniques a chance because you're too busy to see if they work.

Notice a commonality?

They're all lifestyle/mindset perpetuating factors.

CHAPTER EIGHT

Massaging Mom Until One of Us Dies

I thought long and hard about this chapter because it might be the most important one. The other chapters contain the information I wanted to convey, but just providing information alone isn't really my goal.

My goal is to have you actually use the information to improve the quality of your work life and maybe even your life-life. I know you're busy though, and may not have time immediately to do all the experimentation and practice involved in taking this information from the printed page and applying it to the massage room. If that's the case, I want you to remember it and come back to it later. To help you do that, I want to plant my flag in a little corner of your mind by telling you a story that illustrates why extending my massage career has been so important to me:

The room was silent except for the noises coming from the medical devices that were keeping my dad alive in the ICU. He'd taken a big gamble with an elective heart surgery and he was losing the bet. The family sat around him. My mom, who was in a wheelchair, held his hand.

It was time for the big decision; the decision that many have faced or will have to face—should we pull the plug on our loved one?

The saddest part for me wasn't just Dad's death, but also watching Mom struggle to grasp what was happening. Mom's ability to comprehend wasn't what it used to be. She'd had a stroke. She was different. She forgot things. She got confused.

Unlike Lisa and I who could calculate the risks of surgery and prepare ourselves for the worst-case scenario, Mom couldn't. Yesterday her husband had her looked her in the eye and said "I love you." Now a pinging machine was the only indicator that he was still—technically—alive.

I was worried about how she'd handle the sudden, unexpected death of her life partner, and promised myself that I'd fight to stay connected to her. To do that, I fell back on one of the things that had connected us for decades: Massage.

I'd started training to be a massage therapist in 1992 and as with most schools at the time, most of the massage practice happened outside of the classroom. My mom happily volunteered to be my first "massage body" to practice on.

I have to admit that she was good at getting a massage. She had no problem telling me if I was on the right spot, or if I was pressing too hard, or if it felt good. And she really appreciated my work, especially since she had post-polio syndrome.

It was a good arrangement and we both got what we wanted: She got some pain relief and an opportunity to connect with her wayward son, and I got my massage certification. In my mind, once I was no longer a student, it was time to say goodbye to "practice clients" and move on to paying clients. *Thanks for the help though, Mama!* But she wasn't having it.

"I want to be one of your paying customers now."

You do?

"Yes. Once a week."

Once a week? For how long?

"Until one of us dies."

Fast forward to September 15th, 2015. My mom climbed onto my table as she had for 23 years, except that this time something was profoundly different – the man she had loved and been with for 68 years was gone. Our massage sessions became even more important; a touchstone; a way for us to hold on to each other.

Fast forward again to late 2019. Mom was in a rehab center after a series of health issues and even though she couldn't get on my table any more, I could still massage her arthritic knees. I could still use my hands to say, "It's okay, Mom." And her tired eyes could still answer back, "It's okay, sonny." She passed peacefully shortly after that.

For twenty-seven years, massage had been the vehicle that gave us the opportunity to maintain and strengthen our bond and I hadn't even realized it until she was gone. Can you imagine what we'd have lost out on if pain had ended my massage career early? I don't even want to think about it.

What will *you* lose out on if pain ends your massage career early? I don't want you to have to find out. So if you're in pain but you don't have the bandwidth now, please come back to this book later when you can put in the time necessary to see if it works for you as it did for me.

As I wrapped up my work on this book, I found myself thinking of my friend Xentho. My journey to massaging pain free started with the lesson X taught me about leaning. He'd been my timely teacher—my first sage, if you will.

That made me think of a TV series in the 70s called Kung Fu. David Carradine played Kwai Chang Caine, a Shaolin monk who was referred to as "Grasshopper" by his sage, Master Po. Grasshopper's test—to prove he was ready to leave the monastery—required that he be able to successfully snatch a pebble from Master Po's hand. He passed the test and got the pebble.

Finishing this book without catching up with "Master X" didn't feel right, so I found him on Facebook and we messaged each other. I'm happy to report that at 67, X is still going strong and has massage clients coming out of his ears. We reminisced about old times and then I thanked him for teaching me how to lean.

"Yep," he said. "You falling asleep yet?"

Haha. Yep. Dreaming even.

"Good," he said. "Now you're doing it right."

Finally, I got my pebble.

Afterward

If you'd like to continue your own journey to massaging pain free with me, go to www.painfreemassagetherapist. com. Spoiler alert: There's no pebble for you there. But there will be instructional videos and other helpful information, all free of charge. If you have a question, ask me at mark@ painfreemassagetherapist.com. I'm here to help.

References

1. https://brucelee.com/podcast-blog/2017/9/12/63-research-your-own-experience

2. Edward G. Mohr, CPE, CSP, NCTM, "Proper Body Mechanics from an Engineering Perspective." Ergonomics, Volume 14, Issue 2

3. Edward G. Mohr, CPE, CSP, NCTM, "Proper Body Mechanics from an Engineering Perspective." Ergonomics, Volume 14, Issue 2, p. 148

4. Edward G. Mohr, CPE, CSP, NCTM, "Proper Body Mechanics from an Engineering Perspective." Ergonomics, Volume 14, Issue 2, p. 141

5. Edward G. Mohr, CPE, CSP, NCTM, "Proper Body Mechanics from an Engineering Perspective." Ergonomics, Volume 14, Issue 2, p. 140

6. Edward G. Mohr, CPE, CSP, NCTM, "Proper Body Mechanics from an Engineering Perspective." Ergonomics, Volume 14, Issue 2, p. 145

7. Edward G. Mohr, CPE, CSP, NCTM, "Proper Body Mechanics from an Engineering Perspective." Ergonomics, Volume 14, Issue 2, p. 148

8. https://www.youtube.com/watch?v=asP4qZ0bx4w

9. https://www.youtube.com/watch?v=asP4qZ0bx4w

10. https://www.youtube.com/watch?v=asP4qZ0bx4w

11. Travell & Simons Myofascial Pain and Dysfunction: The Trigger Point Manual, Volume 1, p. 103

12. https://en.wikiquote.org/wiki/Richard_Feynman

Made in United States
North Haven, CT
06 January 2022

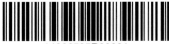

14266595R00091